Supreme Health & Fitness by Sean Ali!

Presents:

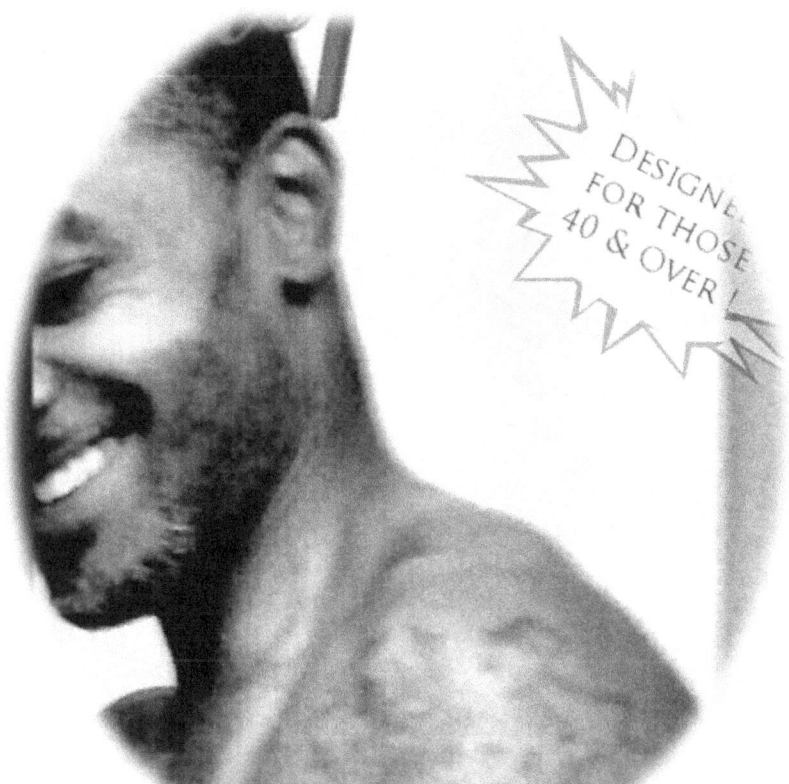

DESIGNE
FOR THOSE
40 & OVER

Enjoying Abundant Life!

Scientific Concepts to Successfully Build Your Supreme Health!

Specifically Designed for those of Us 40 & Over.......But Great for EVERYONE!

ENJOYING ABUNDANT LIFE!

*Scientific Concepts to Successfully Build Your Supreme Health!

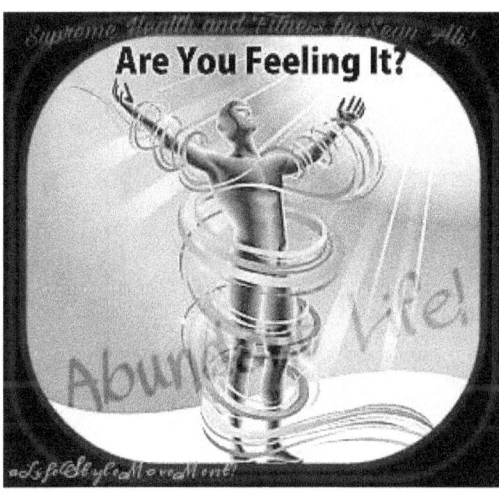

Assisting Scientist:

Khalil Malik * Kareem Tyree * Gabriella Monique

What is Life?

Why do some of us appear more Vital & Alive?

What separates the living from the dead?

Are we born with a certain amount of Vitality, that when it 'runs-out' we die?

Are there ways we can enhance and extend our Vitality & Aliveness?

Supreme Health & Fitness by Sean Ali!

Achieving and Maintaining Supreme Health and Fitness by increasing the level of Knowledge and Science of Life!

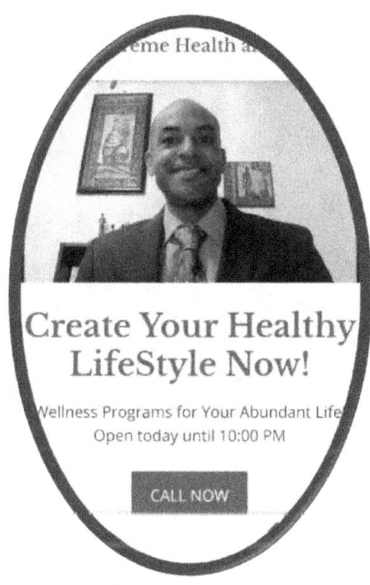

Table of Contents

*****

Introduction

*****

Peace and Blessings of Life!

This book represents Volume 1 of our Abundant Life Series, wherein we attempt to examine Life from a Pathophysiological perspective to discover the Solution to Life Abundant!

As the title expresses, this book is an introduction into the Scientific concepts that form the services and core principles of Supreme Health and Fitness!

✓ Do you have health issues that you want to solve?

✓ Do you want to improve the quality of your life?

✓ Do you want to successfully enjoy your abundant life?

***If you have answered yes to any of these questions than this book is for YOU!

There is only a small and very limited amount of natural ways that we as Humans can die. Even though we all know that we have to eventually make our transition one day, we have the ability to literally die when we want to.....Our Death and LIFE is up to us!!!!

With this book we explore the journey to Successfully Enjoying Abundant Life!

I have found that the first step to abundant life is in answering the question - How Long Do You Want To Live?

Medical Science has compiled a list of all the ways we die. On this list, which we use in this book, they have deduced the top 10 ways that cause our pre-mature death or transition. As morbid as this may seem, the wonderful thing is that we can be Scientist and find where we may be on this list and have the perfect opportunity to Save and Heal Self!

If I can show you HOW to eliminate your Cause of death, then what would you be left with ?

Our basic common denominator is a Cell. Life and Death for us occurs at the Cellular level.

In this small book, we take a closer examination at the Life Cycle of Cells - which we fundamentally ARE = Trillions of Cells!! Looking at our physical body at its basic Root = Cell, makes it infinitely easier to not only accurately develop Solutions, but also the qualifications to Successfully apply them = Supreme Health and Fitness = ABUNDANT LIFE!!

The Human Body is a Perfect Machine! The Heart beats and circulates Life through the Body and the Lungs Inhale the Breath Of Life AUTOMATICALLY! All we have to do is very limited maintenance and we can literally Live ForEver!!

The proper forms and amounts of Energy (Nutrients) intake in combination with an Active/Motion Lifestyle form the foundation of the antithesis of Death.

YES, IT IS THIS EASY !!!!!

Every food decision we make has only 2 possible conclusions = Death or LIFE....meaning that our food is either our Poison or our Medicine.....but there are NO other options. So, when we have access to the best research and data, it allows us to make the Best decisions possible and Create an Atmosphere of LIFE IN SELF!

It's NEVER too late.....But the process doesn't Start until YOU START IT !!!!

Open this book and start the process to Successfully Build YOUR own Supreme Health and ENJOY ABUNDANT LIFE!!!

PEACE!

Sean Ali

Owner & Life Coach

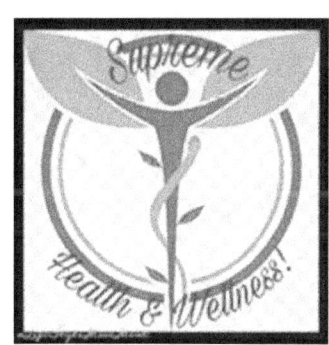

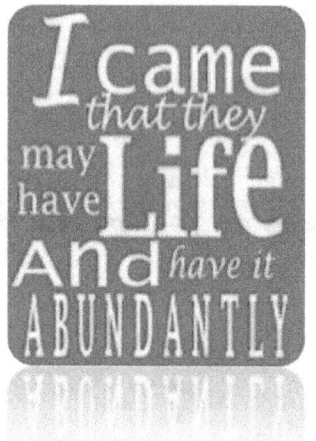

Chapter 1 ......

How Long Do YOU Want To Live?

*****

Have you ever thought about How long you want to live? And now that you have been approached with this question what type of answers do you come up with?

Can you formulate an actual number for the answer? Or can you only say an abstract answer such as - I want to live as long as I can?

The answer to this question is the root foundation of the lifestyle that you will create. If you haven't answered the question or never thought about the question, then the chances of you having an unhealthy lifestyle significantly increase.

Here's another perspective to think about …. Do you like yourself enough to want to extend your life?

Do you love your life to want to take the few necessary measures to preserve it?

If you know that you want to live 200 years, then you will create a lifestyle that will allow you to live 200 years. It's no difference than if you have a 20 year plan and you produce a plan of daily activities to cover that 20 year span, all we are doing is extending your scope and vision.

We can't say that what we can conceive we can achieve it not be able to apply that to answering how long do you want to live.

We cannot have the ability to create a 20 year plan and have the power to move our bodies into fulfilling that and **not** also have this ability and power in creating a 200, 300 or 400 year lifespan and then moving our bodies into for filling it.

There is no mystery to death. The mystery is in life.

When we are looking at health wellness and life and death they are all revolved around your lifestyle.

When we come out of the womb the first lifestyle that we are under is that about what parents or guardians. As we grow and develop, we begin to formulate our own ideas about our own lives and then we incorporate this in create our own lifestyles.

We are all under the law of cause and effect.

And unless you were born with a particular element or disease then it had to be created. When we come out of the womb, we have a perfectly functioning immune system that is specifically created to keep healthy in safe.

So, the only way we can get sick or disease is if we have a compromised immune system.

If you are born with a healthy immune system, how do you compromise it - your lifestyle.

It is your lifestyle that creates your health status. It is your health status that determines the quality of your life and how long you will actually live.

Life and Healing have been made inherently mysterious and as if it is seemingly impossible to have Abundant Life on our own,

To begin the process, it starts by simply Thinking Healthy!

That's right you must start to produce healthy thoughts about yourself and your life. Our bodies are created to follow our thoughts.

Your body doesn't move unless you wanted to move. Abundant life is a physical aspect, we're in your physical body has to be around for you to participate in and enjoy abundant life.

This is the catalyst that causes you to Seek out and Accept a Healthy LifeStyle that's revolved around Living according to our Nature.

You have to WANT Abundant Life in order to Achieve Abundant Life!

Modern science acknowledges that the essential "stuff" of the universe, including the Universe of the Mind and Body, remains essentially unexplained and that the void inside every atom is pulsating with information or unseen intelligence.

Molecular biologists and geneticists locate this intelligence within DNA.

What we understand as Life unfolds as DNA imparts its coded intelligence into a sequence in which Energy and Information are interchanged for the purpose of building Life from Matter.

Unfortunately, there are various actions and reasons that explain why more of us do not make it even to 100 years let alone to the heights of our life-span potential of Abundant or Ever-Lasting Life!

 Nearly all of us experience some type of potentially life-shortening diseases (e.g., heart disease, cancer). While some experts actually believe that the United States' life expectancy will fall dramatically by at least 2 to 5 years in the near future because of OBESITY.

These experts believe that future generations will have shorter and less healthy lives than their parents for the first time in modern history, unless changes are made (Olshansky 2005).

In the United States, the average person life expectancy is 75 years.

There are 2 methods that are used to calculate or determine your age – Chronoligically and Biologically.

Your Chronological Age is calculated or determined as your Actual Age-in-Years from your birth date.

However, what really matters is your Biological Age, which is an estimate of your well-being and general health compared to those of others of your age.

For example, people with health problems at 50 are considered to be biologically older than a healthy and vigorous 70-year-old.

The Lesson to be learned here is for you to take control of your health Sooner = NOW, rather than later.

There are certain Biomarkers of Biological Aging that can let you know whether you are doing Better or Worse than your own Chronological Age.

These markers primarily come from blood testing at a physician's office, but the following are several that you can use as a Self-test on your own:

- Blood pressure

- Blood glucose and cholesterol levels

- Field test for cardiorespiratory fitness (e.g., walking test)

- Muscular strength

- Bone mineral density

- Skin elasticity

- Cognitive abilities, including memory

- Blood markers for systemic inflammation

Biological Age

It is difficult to obtain a definite calculation of your Biological Age. However, if you can answer questions about different health factors, including cholesterol levels, blood pressure, exercise habits, and more, try one of several free online calculators:

- Life Expectancy Calculator available at http://www.livingto100.com

- Real Age Test available at www.realage.com

It is unknown how valid the tests are, but taking either or both of the online tests may point out some ways to change your lifestyle that can improve your health and wellness.

Most of us desire a Long Life; however, let us be mindful of the admonition given by the French essayist, Michel de Montaigne: ***"The usefulness of living lies not in duration but in what you make of it. Some have lived long and lived little."***

Improving our Thought process is intricate in improving our physical Health and Wellness.

Our Minds and Bodies are Related with both equating to LIFE.

The factor of 'WHY' do you want to Improve your Life is just as important as the 'HOW'.

Enjoying Abundant Life begins as easily as a DECISION. We have to decide HOW long that we want to LIVE and act accordingly. THAT SIMPLE......THAT EASY!!

HOW LONG DO YOU WANT TO LIVE?

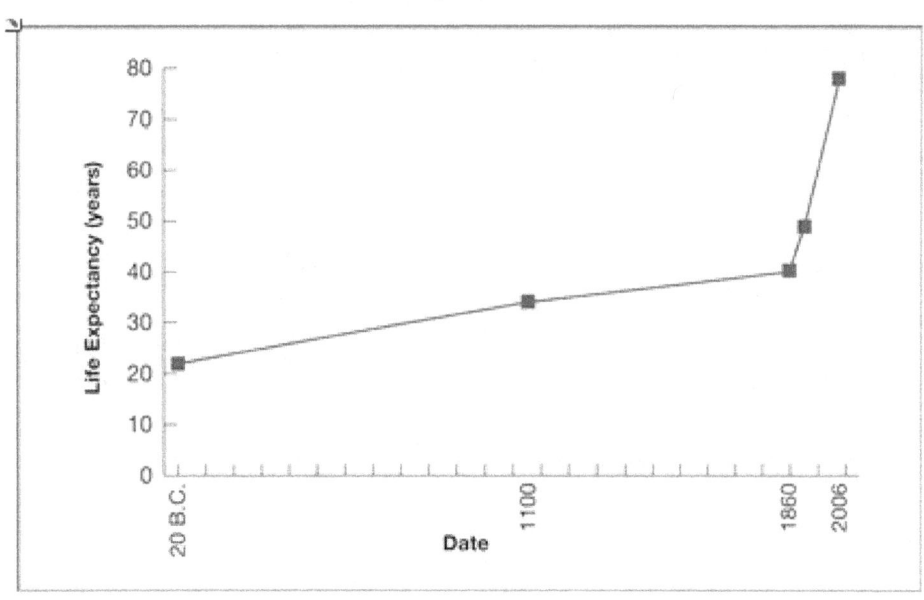

Life expectancy since Julius Caesar.

What Are the Leading Causes of Death?

There are more than 100,000 diseases. However, nearly 60% of the U.S. population dies from just three causes: heart disease, cancer, and stroke. The top 10 causes account for almost 80% of all deaths. Not one of the diseases below the top 10 accounts for even 1% of deaths. Therefore, to live a long and healthy life, the data suggest, that we focus primarily on preventing the top 10 diseases and not the 100,000 others. We go into more detail in Chapter 4.

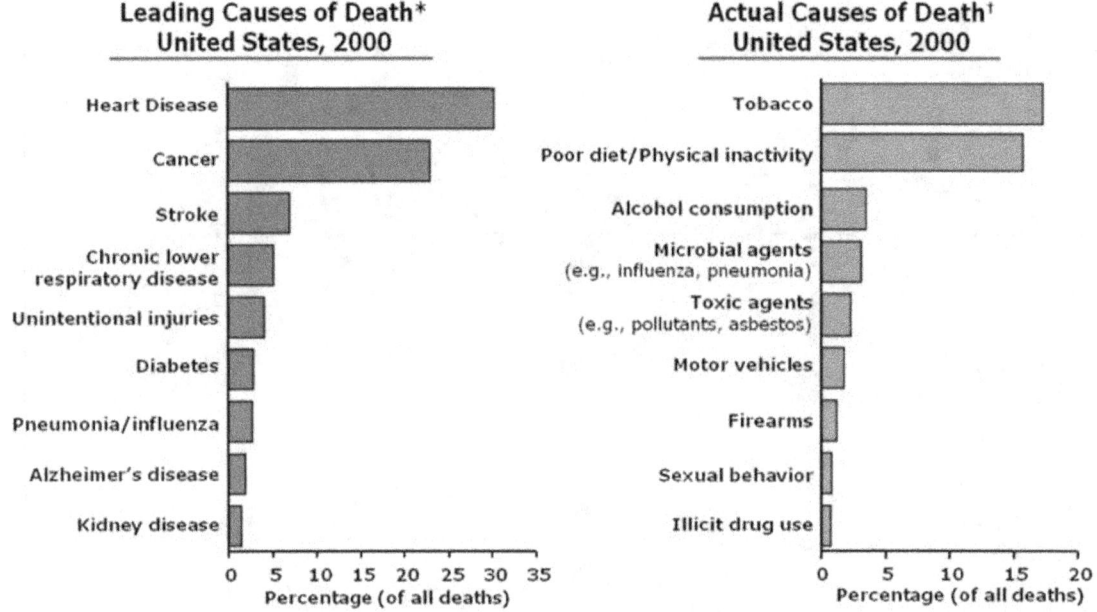

* Miniño AM, Arias E, Kochanek KD, Murphy SL, Smith BL. Deaths: final data for 2000. National Vital Statistics Reports 2002; 50(15):1-120.
† Mokdad AH, Marks JS, Stroup DF, Gerberding JL. Actual causes of death in the United States, 2000. JAMA. 2004;291(10):1238-1246.

What Are the Actual Causes of Death?

What actually kills us?

By answering this question, we can successfully develop services and programs that allow us to not only extend our Life-spans, but significantly improve the Quality of our Lives.

Many people and even health professionals have come up with the answer of heart disease, followed by cancer and stroke—the top three leading causes of death.

Epidemiologists thought that it did not help, when someone died of a heart attack, to conclude

Rank	Actual Cause	Percentage of Deaths
1	Tobacco use	18.1
2	Obesity (inactivity/poor diet)	16.6
3	Alcohol consumption	3.5
4	Microbial agents (flu, pneumonia)	3.1
5	Toxic agents	2.3
6	Motor vehicles	1.8
7	Firearms	1.2
8	Sexual behavior	0.8
9	Illicit drug use	0.7
10	Other	<.05

merely that the cause was disease of the heart. They wanted to know what caused the disease of the heart in the first place, and what caused cancer or the stroke.

They determined that more than half the instances of these diseases were attributable to a handful of largely preventable behaviors: smoking, poor diet, physical inactivity, and alcohol consumption.

Our lifestyle, not our genes, largely determines if and when we suffer from one or more of the top causes of death.

By knowing WHAT can kill us or HOW we die, then it's much easier to Avoid these causes and ENJOY ABUNDANT LIFE!

Over the past four decades, there have been thousands of studies performed that have examined the relationship between physical activity and the risk of various diseases and death. The ***overwhelming*** conclusion is that regular participation in physical activity results in a reduced risk of numerous diseases and death from all causes. ***Regular participation in physical activity reduces the risk of death from all causes by about 40% (relative risk decreased from 1.0 to 0.6).***

Doing physical activity on a regular basis also has been shown to have a similar impact on the following:

• **Cardiorespiratory health**: Physical activity reduces the risk of heart disease and stroke, lowers blood pressure (BP), improves the blood lipid profile, and increases CRF.

• **Metabolic health**: Physical activity reduces the risk of developing type 2 diabetes and helps to control blood glucose in those who already have type 2 diabetes.

• **Musculoskeletal health**: Physical activity slows the loss of bone density that occurs with aging, and it lowers the risk of hip fractures. In addition, it improves pain management in people with arthritis. Finally, progressive muscle-strengthening activities increase or preserve muscle mass, strength, and power

• **Cancer**: Physically active people have a significantly lower risk of colon cancer and breast cancer. In addition, there is some evidence that physical activity reduces the risk of endometrial cancer and lung cancer.

• **Mental health**: Physical activity lowers the risk of depression and age-related cognitive decline, and it improves the quality of sleep.

• **Functional ability and fall prevention**: Physical activity reduces the risk of functional limitations (e.g., ability to do activities of daily living), and for those older adults at risk of falling, physical activity is safe and reduces this risk.

Critical Thinking

1. If I help YOU to Eliminate YOUR Causes of Death ... What are YOU left with??

2. How Long Do You Want To Live??

Progress in the Leading Causes of Death

Death Rates (per 100,000 persons), 2005-2012*

Cause of death	2005	2012	Progress
1.Heart disease	216.8	170.5	Yes
2.Cancers	185.1	166.5	Yes
3.Chronic lower respiratory diseases	43.9	41.5	Insufficient
4.Stroke	48.0	36.9	Yes
5.Unintentional injuries	39.5	39.1	Insufficient
6.Alzheimer's disease	24.0	23.8	Insufficient
7.Diabetes	24.9	21.2	Yes
8.Pneumonia and influenza	21.0	14.4	Yes
9.Kidney disease	14.7	13.1	Yes
10.Suicide	10.9	12.6	No

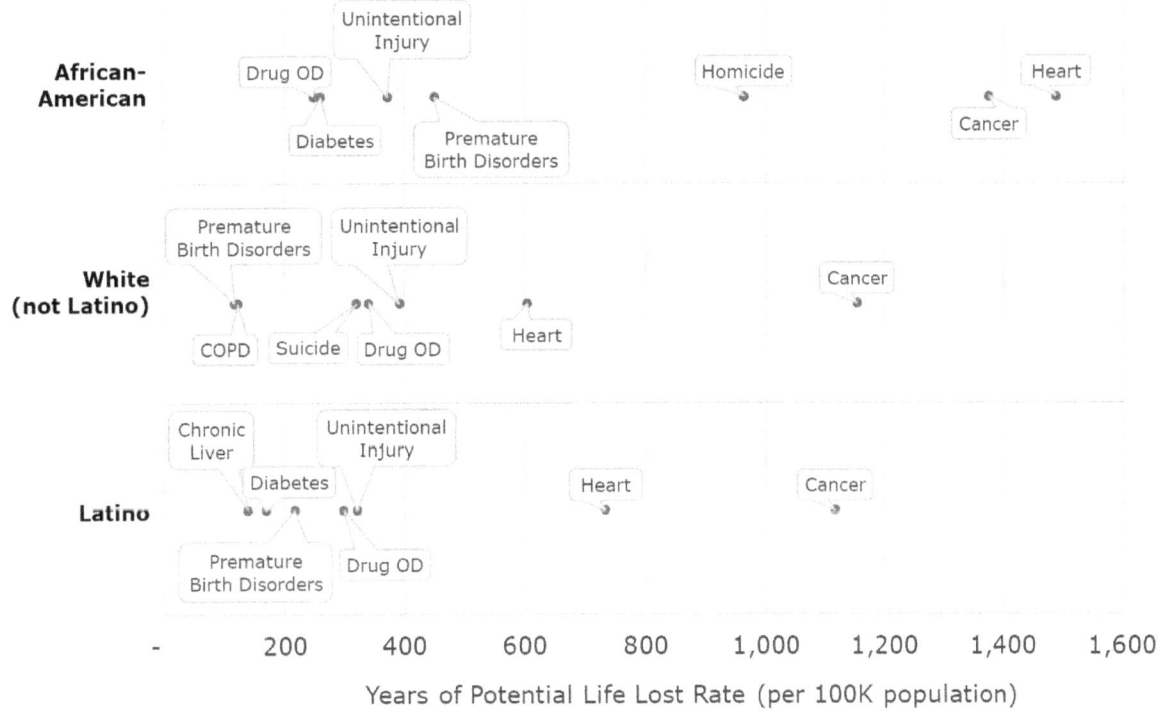

Top causes of years of potential life lost by race/ethnicity (2013-2015)

Chapter 2 ...

Y.P.L.L and Pre-Mature Death

* * * * *

We know that in all industrialized countries, the average life expectancy is 75 years of age. Which means that they expect YOU to live at least 75 years of age. Any death that occurs before the age of 75 is classified under the statistic of YPLL, an acronym that stands for ***Years*** of ***Potential Life Lost***.

This is the statistic that covers premature death.

Understanding this statistic really takes away from any mysterious concepts of death. Understanding the YPLL category removes any illusions or disillusionment about death. Because in order for you to dad before the age of 75 years did you had to significantly damage your biological functions to prohibit them from reproducing life – Your Life.

Do you have a YPLL count??

Are you on your Path to Your Pre-Mature Death ... or the Journey to Your Abundant Life?

Premature Death is a Rate

Rates measure the number of events (i.e., deaths, births, etc.) in a given time period (generally one or more years) divided by the average number of people at risk during that period. Rates help us compare data across counties with different population sizes. All the years of potential life lost in a county during a three-year period are summed and divided by the total population of the county during that same time period.

This value is then multiplied by 100,000 to calculate the years of potential life lost under age 75 per 100,000 people.

Years of potential life lost (YPLL) or potential years of life lost (PYLL), is an estimate of the average years a person would have lived if he or she had not died prematurely. It is, therefore, a measure of premature mortality.

As an alternative to death rates, it is a method that gives more weight to deaths that occur among younger people. An alternative is to consider the effects of both disability and premature death using disability adjusted life years.

This measure is used to help quantify social and economic loss owing to premature death, and it has been promoted to emphasize specific causes of death affecting younger age groups.

YPLL inherently incorporates age at death, and its calculation mathematically weights the total deaths by applying values to death at each age.

YPLL Calculation

To calculate the years of potential life lost, the analyst has to set an upper reference age.

The reference age should correspond roughly to the life expectancy of the population under study.

In the developed world, this is commonly set at age 75, but it is essentially arbitrary.

YPLL can be calculated using individual level data or using age grouped data.[2]

Briefly, for the individual method, each person's YPLL is calculated by subtracting the person's age at death from the reference age.

If a person is older than the reference age when he or she dies, that person's YPLL is set to zero (i.e., there are no "negative" YPLLs).

In effect, only those who die before the reference age are included in the calculation.

Some examples:

i.   Reference age = 75; Age at death = 60; YPLL[75] = 75 − 60 = 15

ii.   Reference age = 75; Age at death = 6 months; YPLL[75] = 75 − 0.5 = 74.5

iii.   Reference age = 75; Age at death = 80; YPLL[75] = 0 (age at death greater than reference age)

To calculate the YPLL for a particular population in a particular year, the analyst sums the individual YPLLs for all individuals in that population who died in that year. This can be done for all-cause mortality or for cause-specific mortality.

Person-years of potential life lost in the United States in 2016

Cause of premature death	Person-years lost
Cancer	8,628,000 person-years
Heart disease and strokes	8,760,000 person-years
Accidents and other injuries	5,873,000 person-years
All other causes	13,649,000 person-years

Understanding this statistic or category should open the door for you to be able to expand what you consider old age to be.

It should also help you to answer the question on how long do you want to live.

Right now, you are expected to live to at least 75 years of age.

Are you on path to do that right now?

The determining factor to whether we reach 75 years of life or suffer premature death is our lifestyle.

The only other exception is if you were born with a hereditary predisposition that causes premature death.

If you do not have a genetic predisposition, then your body is created to grow and develop.

And when a body dies, they complete an autopsy to determine the Cause Of Death …. Because death is NOT Natural…. It has to be Caused.

And it is your lifestyle that is the Cause of your pre-mature death.

The purpose of this book is to introduce scientific concepts so -that we can realistically conceive and plan our life-span ….. And once we have a realistic plan then we can realistically execute it and Successfully Achieve and Enjoy Abundant Life!

Table 2. Actual Causes of Death in the United States in 1990 and 2000

Actual Cause	No. (%) in 1990*	No. (%) in 2000
Tobacco	400 000 (19)	435 000 (18.1)
Poor diet and physical inactivity	300 000 (14)	400 000 (16.6)
Alcohol consumption	100 000 (5)	85 000 (3.5)
Microbial agents	90 000 (4)	75 000 (3.1)
Toxic agents	60 000 (3)	55 000 (2.3)
Motor vehicle	25 000 (1)	43 000 (1.8)
Firearms	35 000 (2)	29 000 (1.2)
Sexual behavior	30 000 (1)	20 000 (0.8)
Illicit drug use	20 000 (<1)	17 000 (0.7)
Total	**1 060 000** (50)	**1 159 000** (48.2)

*Data are from McGinnis and Foege.[1] The percentages are for all deaths.

Cause of disparity in rate of years of potential life lost African-American vs. white (not Latino)

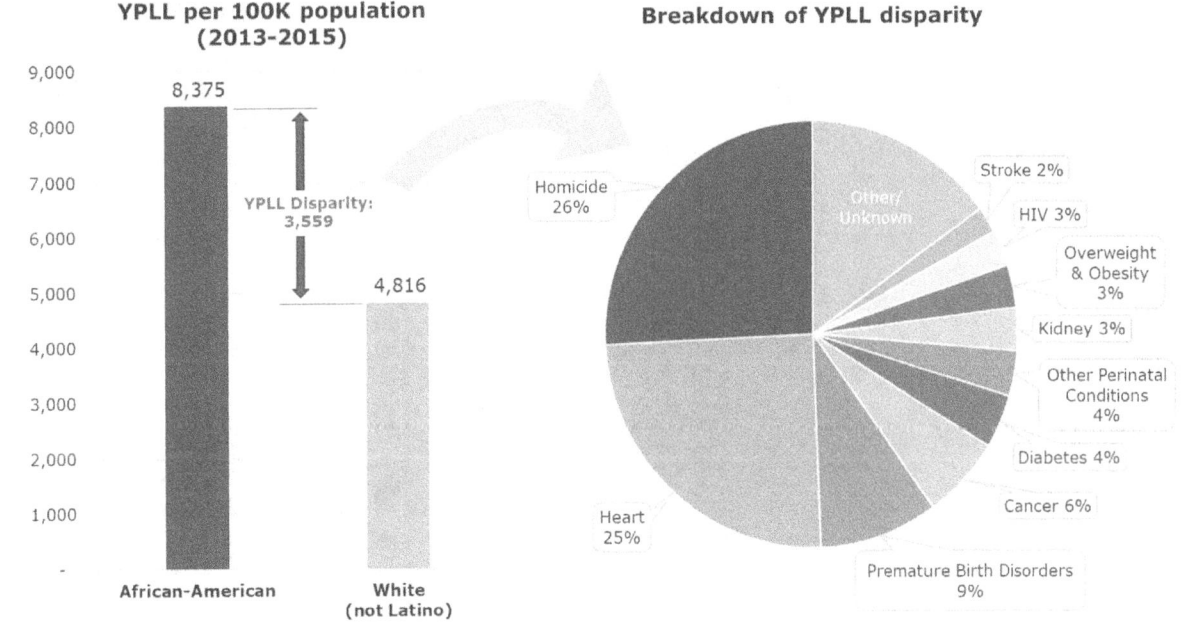

YPLL per 100K population
(2013-2015)

Breakdown of YPLL disparity

Chapter 3 ....

What is Dis-Ease?

*****

Disease is defined as a Structural or Functional Change in the Body that is harmful to the Organism.

A **disease** is a particular abnormal condition that negatively affects the structure or function of part or all of an organism, and that is not due to any external injury.

Diseases are often construed as **medical conditions** that are associated with specific symptoms and signs. A disease may be caused by external factors such as pathogens or by internal dysfunctions.

As an example, internal dysfunctions of the immune system can produce a variety of different diseases, including various forms of immunodeficiency, hypersensitivity, allergies and autoimmune disorders.

In Us, *disease* is often used more broadly to refer to any condition that causes pain, dysfunction, distress, social problems, or death to the person afflicted, or similar problems for those in contact with the person. In this broader sense, it sometimes includes injuries, disabilities, disorders, syndromes, infections, isolated symptoms, deviant behaviors, and atypical variations of structure and function, while in other contexts and for other purposes these may be considered distinguishable categories. Diseases can affect people not only physically, but also mentally, as contracting and living with a disease can alter the affected person's perspective on life.

Death due to disease is what they call death by **natural** causes.

There are four main types of disease: **infectious** diseases, **deficiency** diseases, hereditary diseases (including both genetic diseases and non-genetic hereditary diseases), and **physiological** diseases.

Diseases can also be classified in other ways, such as communicable versus non-communicable diseases.

The deadliest diseases in humans are coronary artery disease (blood flow obstruction), followed by cerebrovascular disease and lower respiratory infections. In developed countries, the diseases that cause the most sickness overall are neuropsychiatric conditions, such as depression and anxiety.

The study of disease is called *pathology*, which includes the study of *etiology*, or cause.

Disease occurs when the Cellular environment changes to such a degree that Tissues are no longer able to perform their normal biological functions and/or maintain it's own life.

For example, with Cataracts, the Crystalline Lens of the Eye undergoes degenerative changes over the course of a person's lifetime and becomes cloudy, obstructing the passage of light and causing decreased visual acuity.

In Diabetes, the extra-cellular Tissue of Blood Vessel walls undergoes changes that lead to narrowing of the Blood Vessels, which in turn leads to decreased Blood Flow, decreased Oxygen delivery, and eventually irreversible damage to Tissues such as the Retina, Skin, Heart, and Kidney.

Both vitamins and minerals help facilitate our structural and our functional properties.

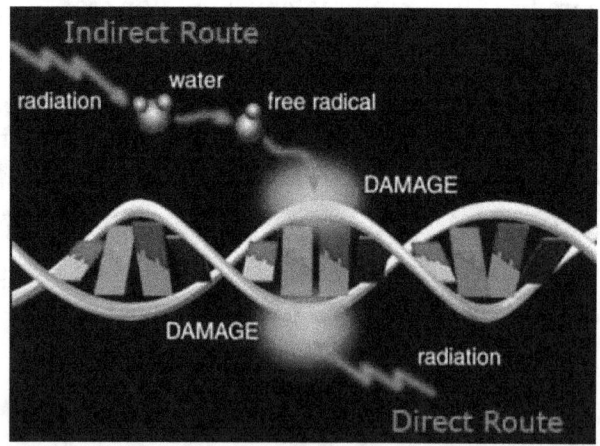

In cancer, mutations accumulating in the Nucleic Acids of Cells result in distorted structure and function of Proteins, which in turn affect the way the Cells interact with or react to other Cells, growth factors, hormones, and the extracellular matrix in their environment.

In multiple sclerosis, destruction of the protective Myelin Sheath around Axons in the Brain results in decreased electrical conduction, which manifests in neurologic signs and symptoms such as weakness, double vision, and incoordination.

In each of these conditions, the ability of Cells or Tissues to optimally perform their function is compromised, with deleterious consequences to the organism.

Also in these cases, disease can easily be described as an INJURY, and by doing so, you change the treatment and therapy.

When you think of disease in its commercial or traditional sense, then you associate medication as the treatment. Medications treat diseases. Our bodies are Earth-based and come from the material of the Earth. This is why food is our building-blocks and medicine.

So, when we are examining a Structural change, this is the Material composition of our body. The treatment or therapy should be Earth-based Solutions.

When we look at a functional change, this would be more indicative of a nutritional issue versus a pharmaceutical therapy.

Manifestations of Disease

We use the term *manifestation* to refer to all the data gathered about a disease as it occurs in a patient. The manifestations that are of interest to the allopathic doctor are symptoms, signs, and laboratory abnormalities

TABLE 2-1 ... Manifestations of Disease

Type of Manifestation	Nature of Data	Name for Collection of Results
Symptoms	Patient's perceptions	History
Signs	Examiner's observations	Physical examination
Laboratory abnormalities	Results of tests and special procedures	Laboratory findings

Symptoms are evidence of disease perceived by the patient, such as pain, a lump, or diarrhea. Health practitioners carefully elicit these during an interview with the patient and record them in the patient's chart as the *history*.

Signs are physical observations made by the person who examines the patient. Examples include tenderness, a mass, or abnormal heart sounds. Signs are elicited and observed during the *physical examination*, the results of which are also recorded in the patient's chart.

Laboratory findings are observations made by the application of tests or special procedures, such as x-rays, blood counts, or biopsies.

Diagnosis is the process of assimilating the information from the history, physical examination, and laboratory findings to identify the condition causing the disease. Diagnosis also refers to the name given to that disease, such as "multiple sclerosis" or "diabetes." This name is a shorthand way of communicating and thinking. It sums up all the essential information from the history, physical examination, and laboratory findings so that an appropriate therapy can be initiated. Underlying diagnosis and treatment is the assumption that diseases of the same name run a predictable course that can be altered, to lesser or greater degree, by medical intervention.

Sometimes a diagnosis cannot immediately be made. As an example, Alzheimer disease cannot be definitively diagnosed until a patient's brain is examined after his or her death. Obviously, it is too late to do anything about it then, so, while the patient is alive, the patient is given a provisional diagnosis of "Alzheimer-type dementia." Other diseases, such as rheumatologic, neurologic, or gastrointestinal ones, may also be vaguely identified (for example, "paralysis of unknown cause") and treated symptomatically until the disease "declares itself," or develops some features that allow its unique identification.

In such cases, the clinical problem—paralysis, dementia—is used as the focus of symptomatic treatment until the patient's disease can be definitively identified.

Syndromes are clusters of findings commonly encountered with more than one disease. As an example, leakage of protein into the urine, low serum protein, and edema are a common set of findings in the "nephrotic syndrome," which can be caused by a number of different diseases that affect the renal glomeruli. The syndrome is a description of a constellation of symptoms, and though treatments can be initiated to alleviate the symptoms and laboratory abnormalities, specific treatment of the disease causing the syndrome is still necessary.

TABLE 2-2 ... Exogenous Causes of Disease

Physical injury

- Trauma

- Heat/cold

- Electricity

- Pressure

- Ionizing radiations

Chemical injury

- Poisoning

- Drug reactions

Microbiologic injury

- Bacteria

- Fungi

- Rickettsiae

- Viruses

- Protozoa

- Helminths

Causes of Disease

Diseases are initiated by injury, which can occur by either external or internal in origin. Agents acting from WITHOUT are termed **Exogenous**; those acting from WITHIN are referred to as **Endogenous**.

Exogenous causes of disease are divided into Physical, Chemical, and Microbiologic (Table 2-2). **Direct Physical** injury is called **Trauma**. Physical Agents causing disease include extremes of heat and cold, electricity, atmospheric pressure changes, and radiation (electromagnetic and particulate).

Chemical injuries are generally subdivided by the manner of injury into ***Poisoning*** (accidental, homicidal, or suicidal) and ***Drug Reactions*** (toxic effects of prescription or proprietary drugs taken to treat disease).

Microbiologic injuries are usually classified by the type of offending organism (bacteria, fungi, rickettsiae, viruses, protozoa, and helminths) and are called **Infections**.

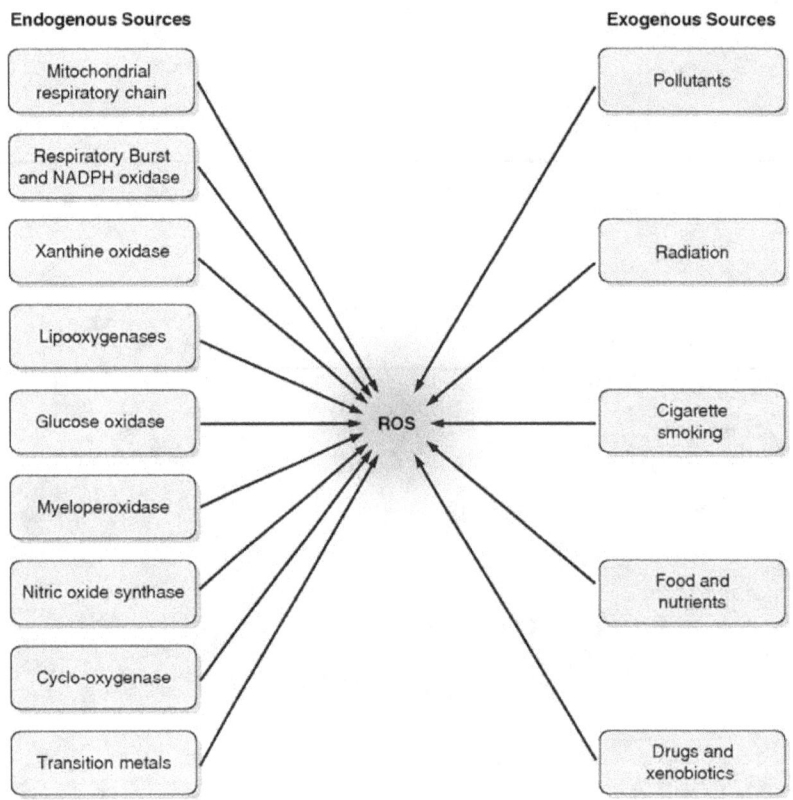

Endogenous causes of disease fall into three large categories (Table 2-3). **Vascular diseases** include obstruction of blood supply to an organ or tissue (e.g., myocardial ischemia secondary to atherosclerosis), hemorrhage (e.g., a ruptured abdominal aortic aneurysm), or altered blood flow (e.g., microvascular changes in diabetes or hypertension).

Immunologic diseases are those caused by aberrations of the immune system. Failure of the immune system to work when it is needed results in immunodeficiency disease.

Overreaction of the immune system causes allergic, or hypersensitivity, diseases. Abnormal reaction of the immune system to endogenous substances causes autoimmune diseases.

The category of **metabolic diseases** encompasses a wide variety of biochemical disorders that may be genetically determined or secondary effects of acquired disease. Metabolic diseases are most commonly categorized as abnormalities primarily involving lipids, carbohydrates, proteins, minerals, vitamins, and fluids.

TABLE 2-3 ... Endogenous Causes of Disease

Vascular
• Obstruction
• Bleeding
• Deranged flow

Immunologic
• Immune deficiency
• Allergy
• Autoimmunity

Metabolic
• Abnormal metabolism or deficiency of:
Lipids
Carbohydrates
Proteins
Minerals
Vitamins
Fluids

Concepts of Disease

In many cases, terms such as *disease*, *disorder*, *morbidity*, *sickness* and *illness* are used interchangeably.

There are situations, however, when specific terms are considered preferable.

Disease: The term *disease* broadly refers to any condition that impairs the normal functioning of the body. For this reason, diseases are associated with dysfunctioning of the body's normal homeostatic processes. The term is used to refer specifically to infectious diseases, which are clinically evident diseases that result from the presence of pathogenic microbial agents, including viruses, bacteria, fungi, protozoa, multicellular organisms, and aberrant proteins known as prions. An infection or colonization that does not and will not produce clinically evident impairment of normal functioning, such as the presence of the normal bacteria and yeasts in the gut, or of a passenger virus, is not considered a disease. By contrast, an infection that is asymptomatic during its incubation period, but expected to produce symptoms later, is usually considered a disease. Non-infectious diseases are all other diseases, including most forms of cancer, heart disease, and genetic disease.

Acquired disease: An acquired disease is one that began at some point during one's lifetime, as opposed to disease that was already present at birth, which is congenital disease. *Acquired* sounds like it could mean "caught via contagion", but it simply means acquired sometime after birth.

Acute disease: An acute disease is one of a short-term nature (acute); the term sometimes also connotes a fulminant nature

Chronic condition or chronic disease: A chronic disease is one that persists over time, often characterized as at least six months but may also include illnesses that are expected to last for the entirety of one's natural life.

Congenital disorder or congenital disease: A congenital disorder is one that is present at birth. It is often a genetic disease or disorder and can be inherited. It can also be the result of a vertically transmitted infection from the mother, such as HIV/AIDS.

Genetic disease: A genetic disorder or disease is caused by one or more genetic mutations. It is often inherited, but some mutations are random and de novo.

Hereditary or inherited disease: A hereditary disease is a type of genetic disease caused by genetic mutations that are hereditary (and can run in families)

Iatrogenic disease: An iatrogenic disease or condition is one that caused by medical intervention, whether as a side effect of a treatment or as an inadvertent outcome.

Idiopathic disease: An idiopathic disease has an unknown cause or source. As medical science has advanced, many diseases with entirely unknown causes have had some aspects of their sources explained and therefore shed their idiopathic status. For example, when germs were discovered, it became known that they were a cause of infection, but particular germs and diseases had not been linked. In another example, it is known that autoimmunity is the cause of some forms of diabetes mellitus type 1, even though the particular molecular pathways by which it works are not yet understood. It is also common to know certain factors are associated with certain diseases. However, association and causality are two very different phenomena, as a third cause might be producing the disease, as well as an associated phenomenon.

Incurable disease: A disease that cannot be cured. Incurable diseases are not necessarily terminal diseases, and sometimes a disease's symptoms can be treated sufficiently for the disease to have little or no impact on quality of life.

Primary disease: A primary disease is a disease that is due to a root cause of illness, as opposed to secondary disease, which is a sequela, or complication that is caused by the primary disease. For example, a common cold is a primary disease, where rhinitis is a possible secondary disease, or sequela. A doctor must determine what primary disease, a cold or a bacterial infection, is causing a patient's secondary rhinitis when deciding whether or not to prescribe antibiotics.

Secondary disease: A secondary disease is a disease that is a sequela or complication of a prior, causal disease, which is referred to as the primary disease or simply the underlying cause (root cause). For example, a bacterial infection can be primary, wherein a healthy person is exposed to a bacteria and becomes infected, or it can be secondary to a primary cause, that predisposes the body to infection. For example, a primary viral infection that weakens the immune system could lead to a secondary bacterial infection. Similarly, a primary burn that creates an open wound could provide an entry point for bacteria, and lead to a secondary bacterial infection.

Terminal disease: A terminal disease is one that is expected to have the inevitable result of death. Previously, AIDS was a terminal disease; it is now incurable, but can be managed indefinitely using medications.

Illness: The terms *illness* and *sickness* are both generally used as synonyms for *disease*. However, the term *illness* is occasionally used to refer specifically to the patient's personal experience of his or her disease. In this model, it is possible for a person to have a disease without being ill (to have an objectively definable, but asymptomatic, medical condition, such as a subclinical infection, or to have a clinically apparent physical impairment but not feel sick or distressed by it), and to be *ill* without being *diseased* (such as when a person perceives a normal experience as a medical condition, or medicalizes a non-disease situation in his or her life—for example, a person who feels unwell as a result of embarrassment, and who interprets those feelings as sickness rather than normal emotions). Symptoms of illness are often not directly the result of infection, but a collection of evolved responses—sickness behavior by the body—that helps clear infection and promote recovery. Such aspects of illness can include lethargy, depression, loss of appetite, sleepiness, hyperalgesia, and inability to concentrate.

Disorder: A disorder is a functional abnormality or disturbance. Medical disorders can be categorized into mental disorders, physical disorders, genetic disorders, emotional and behavioral disorders, and functional disorders. The term *disorder* is often considered more value-neutral and less stigmatizing than the terms *disease* or *illness*, and therefore is a preferred terminology in some circumstances. In mental health, the term *mental disorder* is used as a way of acknowledging the complex interaction of biological, social, and psychological factors in psychiatric conditions. However, the term *disorder* is also used in many other areas of medicine, primarily to identify physical disorders that are not caused by infectious organisms, such as metabolic disorders.

Medical condition: A **medical condition** is a broad term that includes all diseases, lesions, disorders, or non-pathologic condition that normally receives medical treatment, such as pregnancy or childbirth. While the term *medical condition* generally includes mental illnesses, in some contexts the term is used specifically to denote any illness, injury, or disease except for mental illnesses.

The Diagnostic and Statistical Manual of Mental Disorders (DSM), the widely used psychiatric manual that defines all mental disorders, uses the term *general medical condition* to refer to all diseases, illnesses, and injuries except for mental disorders. This usage is also commonly seen in the psychiatric literature. Some health insurance policies also define a *medical condition* as any illness, injury, or disease except for psychiatric illnesses.

As it is more value-neutral than terms like *disease*, the term *medical condition* is sometimes preferred by people with health issues that they do not consider deleterious. On the other hand, by emphasizing the medical nature of the condition, this term is sometimes rejected, such as by proponents of the autism rights movement.

The term *medical condition* is also a synonym for *medical state*, in which case it describes an individual patient's current state from a medical standpoint. This usage appears in statements that describe a patient as being *in critical condition*, for example.

Morbidity (from Latin *morbidus*, meaning 'sick, unhealthy') is a diseased state, disability, or poor health due to any cause. The term may be used to refer to the existence of any form of disease, or to the degree that the health condition affects the patient. Among severely ill patients, the level of morbidity is often measured by ICU scoring systems. Comorbidity is the simultaneous presence of two or more medical conditions, such as schizophrenia and substance abuse.

In epidemiology and actuarial science, the term "morbidity rate" can refer to either the incidence rate, or the prevalence of a disease or medical condition. This measure of sickness is contrasted with the mortality rate of a condition, which is the proportion of people dying during a given time interval.

Morbidity rates are used in actuarial professions, such as health insurance, life insurance and long-term care insurance, to determine the correct premiums to charge to customers. Morbidity rates help insurers predict the likelihood that an insured will contract or develop any number of specified diseases.

Pathosis or pathology: *Pathosis* (plural *pathoses*) is synonymous with *disease*. The word *pathology* also has this sense, in which it is commonly used by physicians in the medical literature, although some editors prefer to reserve *pathology* to its other senses.

Syndrome: A syndrome is the association of several medical signs, symptoms, or other characteristics that often occur together. Some syndromes, such as Down syndrome, have only one cause. Others, such as Parkinsonian syndrome, have multiple possible causes. For example, acute coronary syndrome is not a single disease itself, but rather the manifestation of any of several diseases, such as myocardial infarction secondary to coronary artery disease. In yet other syndromes, the cause is unknown. A familiar syndrome name often remains in use even after an underlying cause has been found, or when there are a number of different possible primary causes. Examples of the first-mentioned type are that Turner syndrome and DiGeorge syndrome are still often called by the "syndrome" name despite that they can also be viewed as disease entities and not solely as sets of signs and symptoms.

Diseases by Body System

Mental

Mental illness is a broad, generic label for a category of illnesses that may include affective or emotional instability, behavioral dysregulation, cognitive dysfunction or impairment.

Specific illnesses known as mental illnesses include major depression, generalized anxiety disorders, schizophrenia, and attention deficit hyperactivity disorder, to name a few.

Mental illness can be of biological (e.g., anatomical, chemical, or genetic) or psychological (e.g., trauma or conflict) origin. It can impair the affected person's ability to work or study and can harm interpersonal relationships. The term insanity is used technically as a legal term.

Organic

An organic disease is one caused by a physical or physiological change to some tissue or organ of the body. The term sometimes excludes infections. It is commonly used in contrast with mental disorders.

It includes emotional and behavioral disorders if they are due to changes to the physical structures or functioning of the body, such as after a stroke or a traumatic brain injury, but not if they are due to psychosocial issues.

Disease Stages

In an infectious disease, the incubation period is the time between infection and the appearance of symptoms. The latency period is the time between infection and the ability of the disease to spread to another person, which may precede, follow, or be simultaneous with the appearance of symptoms.

Some viruses also exhibit a dormant phase, called viral latency, in which the virus hides in the body in an inactive state. For example, varicella zoster virus causes chickenpox in the acute phase; after recovery from chickenpox, the virus may remain dormant in nerve cells for many years, and later cause herpes zoster (shingles).

Acute disease

An acute disease is a short-lived disease, like the common cold.

Chronic disease

A chronic disease is one that lasts for a long time, usually at least six months. During that time, it may be constantly present, or it may go into remission and periodically relapse. A chronic disease may be stable (does not get any worse) or it may be progressive (gets worse over time). Some chronic diseases can be permanently cured. Most chronic diseases can be beneficially treated, even if they cannot be permanently cured.

Clinical disease

One that has clinical consequences; in other words, the stage of the disease that produces the characteristic signs and symptoms of that disease.[19] AIDS is the clinical disease stage of HIV infection.

Cure

A cure is the end of a medical condition or a treatment that is very likely to end it, while remission refers to the disappearance, possibly temporarily, of symptoms. Complete remission is the best possible outcome for incurable diseases.

Flare-up

A flare-up can refer to either the recurrence of symptoms or an onset of more severe symptoms.

Progressive disease

Progressive disease is a disease whose typical natural course is the worsening of the disease until death, serious debility, or organ failure occurs. Slowly progressive diseases are also chronic diseases; many are also degenerative diseases. The opposite of progressive disease is *stable disease* or *static disease*: a medical condition that exists, but does not get better or worse.

Refractory disease

A refractory disease is a disease that resists treatment, especially an individual case that resists treatment more than is normal for the specific disease in question.

Subclinical disease

Also called **silent disease**, **silent stage**, or **asymptomatic disease**. This is a stage in some diseases before the symptoms are first noted.[20]

Terminal phase

If a person will die soon from a disease, regardless of whether that disease typically causes death, then the stage between the earlier disease process and active dying is the terminal phase.

Extent of Disease

Localized disease

A localized disease is one that affects only one part of the body, such as athlete's foot or an eye infection.

Disseminated disease

A disseminated disease has spread to other parts; with cancer, this is usually called metastatic disease.

Systemic disease

A systemic disease is a disease that affects the entire body, such as influenza or high blood pressure.

Types of Causes

Airborne

An airborne disease is any disease that is caused by pathogens and transmitted through the air.

Foodborne

Foodborne illness or food poisoning is any illness resulting from the consumption of food contaminated with pathogenic bacteria, toxins, viruses, prions or parasites.

Infectious

Infectious diseases, also known as transmissible diseases or communicable diseases, comprise clinically evident illness (i.e., characteristic medical signs or symptoms of disease) resulting from the infection, presence and growth of pathogenic biological agents in an individual host organism. Included in this category are *contagious diseases*—an infection, such as influenza or the common cold, that commonly spreads from one person to another—and *communicable diseases*—a disease that can spread from one person to another, but does not necessarily spread through everyday contact.

Lifestyle

A lifestyle disease is any disease that appears to increase in frequency as countries become more industrialized and people live longer, especially if the risk factors include behavioral choices like a sedentary lifestyle or a diet high in unhealthful foods such as refined carbohydrates, trans fats, or alcoholic beverages.

Non-communicable

A non-communicable disease is a medical condition or disease that is non-transmissible. Non-communicable diseases cannot be spread directly from one person to another. Heart disease and cancer are examples of non-communicable diseases in humans.

Leading causes of death in perspective

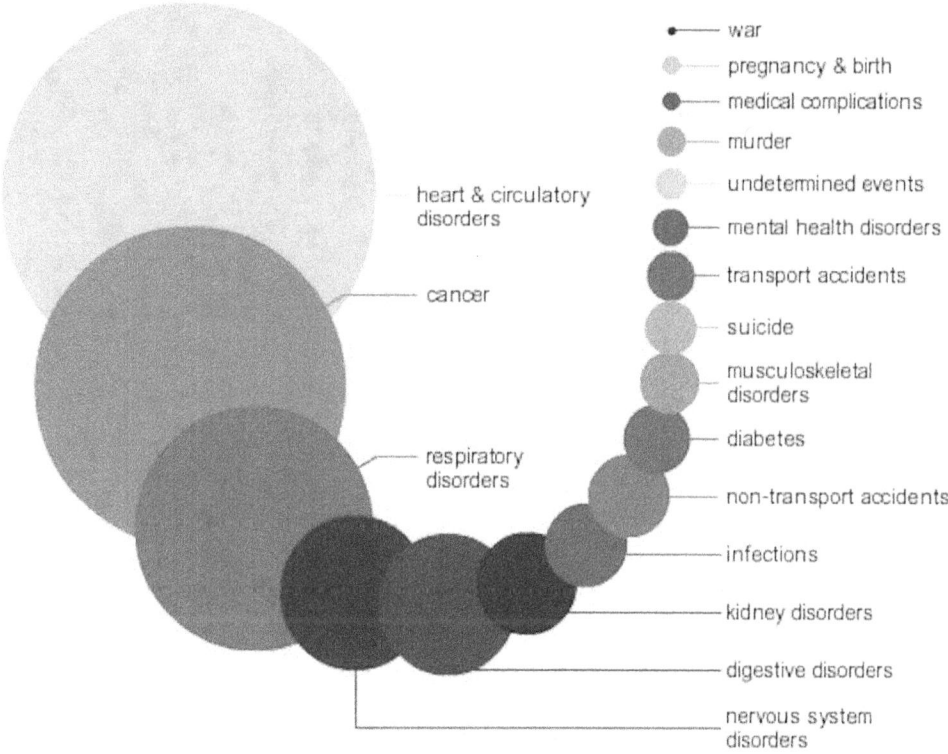

Chapter 4 ....

Causes Of Death - Mortality

*****

Causes of Death is also referred to as **Mortality** and is a list that's largely compiled by government agencies from death certificates, filled out by trained personnel at the time of a person's death.

Approximately 70% of all deaths in the United States are accounted for by the five most frequent causes. When we are looking at the causes of death they are all classified as controllable and or preventable. This means that you either caused the imbalance or you interfered with your body seeking to achieve that balance.

The causes of death vary considerably by age.

TABLE 3–1 Overall Leading Causes of Death, United States, 2016

Cause of Death	Number of Deaths
1. Heart disease	596,339
2. Cancer	575,313
3. Chronic pulmonary disease	143,382
4. Cerebrovascular disease (stroke)	128,931
5. Accidents	122,777
6. Alzheimer dementia	84,691
7. Diabetes	73,282
8. Pneumonia and influenza	53,667
9. Kidney disease	45,731
10. Suicide	38,285
11. Septicemia	35,539
12. Chronic liver disease	33,539
13. Hypertension	27,477
14. Parkinson disease	23,107
15. Pneumonitis due to aspiration	18,090
— all other causes	512,723

Heart disease accounted for 25% of deaths in the United States in 2011 (with this total significantly RISING by 2017) .

The vast majority of these deaths are caused by **Atherosclerosis**, which is a classified as a degenerative disease of Arteries.

Let's take a moment and examine the **controllable** and **preventable** part of the causes of death and use atherosclerosis as an example. We see that it is classified as a degenerative **disease**. When most people see the word **disease**, they think that it is something caused from an **external** source. But it is in fact an internal cause.

You have to both - eat the wrong foods and lead a sedentary lifestyle .

Cholesterol is a main element of the material that clogs your arteries. The only food source that cholesterol comes from is animal meats and products. This is the material that forms the plaque or build up.

Note: There are no good food sources of cholesterol …. We do not need any cholesterol in our diets ….. There are good or bad cholesterol levels within in your body.

On the other hand, you are not exercising enough so your blood is moving so slow that this material has a chance to collect and build up informed the plaque.

Completely controllable and preventable.

And this is not a pharmaceutical therapy or solution because if you continue to eat the wrong foods and continue to lead a sedentary lifestyle - then you will continue to have plaque buildup.

Over the course of many years these lipid-rich deposits develop in the Arterial Lining.

These areas of thickening may induce the sudden development of a thrombus that completely occludes the vessel and obstructs the flow of blood to a portion of myocardium (heart muscle), which subsequently dies.

This is a "heart attack," or myocardial infarct.

Myocardial infarcts are more frequent and occur at an earlier age in men than in women under the age of 50, but after this the incidence of myocardial infarct equalizes between the two sexes.

Myocardial infarcts can be lethal by causing sudden death (death within an hour of the onset of symptoms), or they can induce degenerative and compensatory changes in the heart that can be lethal from days to years after the infarct, such as sudden rupture of the myocardial wall or congestive heart failure

The most common causes of death of children aged 1–14 years are given in Table 3–2. In children less than 1 year, the most common causes of death relate to congenital anomalies, low birth weight, and complications of premature birth.

TABLE 3–2 … Leading Causes of Death in Children Aged 1–14 Years, United States, 2016

Cause of Death	Number of Deaths
1. Accidental trauma	3,868
2. Cancer	1,284
3. Congenital anomalies	859
4. Homicide	756
5. Heart disease	314
6. Sepsis	172
7. Influenza and pneumonia	149
8. Cerebrovascular disease	165
9. Benign neoplasms	136
10. Chronic lower respiratory disease	119

TABLE 3–3 … Leading Causes of Disability Among Adults and Percentage of All Disabilities

Condition	Percentage
Arthritis	19
Back and spine problems	17
Heart trouble	7
Mental or emotional problems	5
Lung, respiratory trouble	5
Diabetes	4.5
Deafness or hearing problems	4
Stiffness or deformity of limbs/extremities	4
Blindness	3
Stroke	2

TABLE 3–4 …. Top 20 Reasons for Office Visits to a Physician in the United States

1. Routine infant or child health check

2. Hypertension

3. Acute upper respiratory infections

4. Arthritis and related conditions

5. Diabetes

6. Spinal disorders

7. Specific procedures

8. Malignant neoplasms

9. Normal pregnancy

10. Rheumatism

11. Gynecologic examination

12. Otitis media

13. Follow-up examination

14. General medical examination

15. Nonischemic heart disease

16. Sinusitis

17. Allergic rhinitis

18. Ischemic heart disease

19. Asthma

20. Cataracts

Critical Thinking

1. If I help YOU to Eliminate YOUR Causes of Death ... What are YOU left with??

2. How Long Do You Want To Live??

Chapter 5 ...

Cellular Injury, Inflammation & REPAIR!

*****

Review of Structure and Function

Our body is literally comprised up of Cells and intercellular substances that are capable of undergoing dynamic change to carry out body functions, including self-renewal. One or several of the more than 100 Cell types, along with appropriate intercellular substances, make up a tissue.

The term **tissue** is typically used to refer to a functional grouping of Cells and inter-cellular substances.

An **Organ** is one or more Tissues arranged into a structure that carries out a major body function. For an example let's examine the Liver – Liver Tissue forms one massive organ which we in-turn call the Liver, whereas loose connective tissue is a general type of tissue that may be a part of many organs.

The Cells that carry out the main function of an organ, and are usually most abundant and often unique to the organ, are called **Parenchymal** cells.

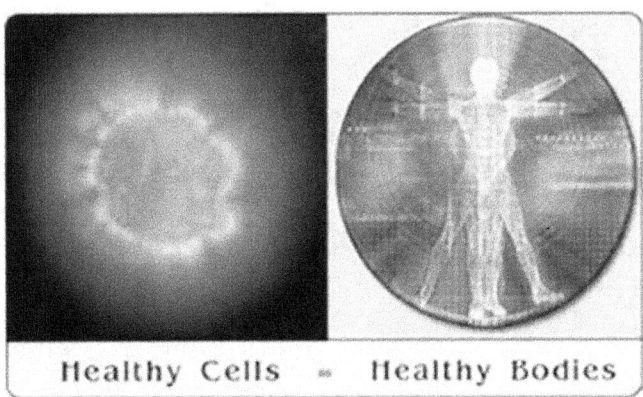

Healthy Cells ≈ Healthy Bodies

Understanding our Cellular Life – Growth, Repair and Death cycles and prepare us to make the best Nutritional and Exercise choices that allow us to successfully Build and Maintain our own Supreme Health and Fitness = Abundant Life!

The Cytoplasm of a Cell contains **Cytoplasmic Organelles**, with specialized functions, and a soluble component called the Cytosol. The Cytoplasm is enclosed by a highly specialized **Cell Membrane** that protects the Cell from physical injury and selectively regulates the entrance and exit of various Ions and Nutrients, including Amino Acids, Sugars, Electrolytes such as Sodium, Potassium, and Calcium, and fluid.

 Movement of Water to and from the Cell is largely dependent on the movement of Ions across the Cell Membrane. A large amount of a Cell's Energy is spent on actively maintaining an Electrical and Osmotic Gradient across the Cell Membrane and maintaining precise control over Intracellular pH, Osmolality, Electrolyte concentration, and fluid balance.

Cytoplasmic organelles include structures such as **Mitochondria**, rough and smooth **Endoplasmic Reticulum**, **Golgi Apparatus**, and **Lysosomes**. Mitochondria are complex, membranous structures that generate Energy for use by the Cell. Injuries that interfere with Energy production often cause the Mitochondria to swell and later condense.

A simple classification of tissue components is shown in Table 4–1. The two most varied classes of cells are Epithelial Cells and Connective Tissue Cells. ***The distinction between these two classes of cells is very important in pathology because they react quite differently in disease situations***.

Epithelial cells work with each other as coherent units to carry out specialized functions, such as protection of body surfaces, secretion of specific products, and special metabolic functions.

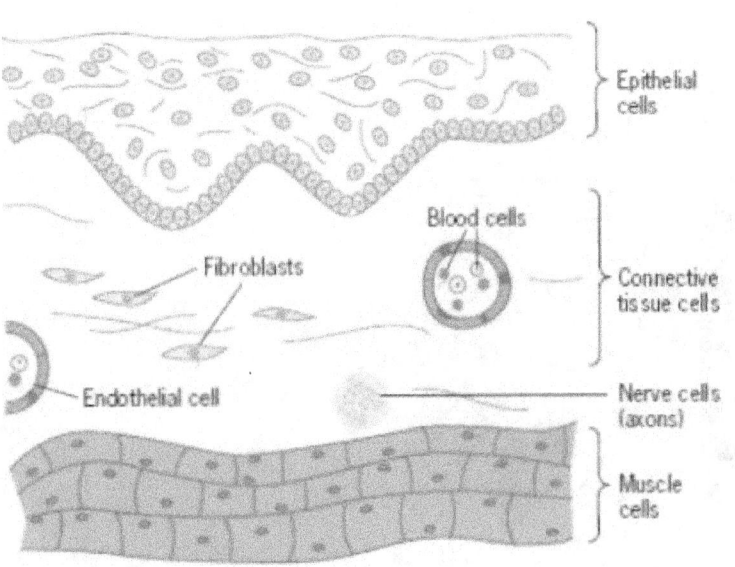

Epithelial cells

Blood cells

Fibroblasts

Connective tissue cells

Endothelial cell

Nerve cells (axons)

Muscle cells

Injury interferes with their specialized function and causes them to revert to a more primitive stage for purposes of reproduction to replace cells that have been killed.

Connective Tissue Cells are more loosely arranged and are involved in general support functions, such as providing physical support and facilitating the movement of fluids and nutrients

Structural Elements of Tissues

Cells

• Epithelium (e.g., mucosal cells of the gastrointestinal tract, epidermis of skin)

• Connective tissue cells

• Fixed: Fibrocytes, chondrocytes, osteocytes, endothelial cells

• Mobile: Blood cells

• Muscle cells (e.g., skeletal muscle, cardiac muscle, smooth muscle of uterus, gastrointestinal tract, bladder)

• Nervous tissue cells

Intercellular substances

• Basement membranes

• Ground substance

• Collagen

• Elastin

• Cartilage

• Bone

NECROSIS	APOPTOSIS
"Accidental"	"Programmed"
Usually affects large areas of contiguous cells	Usually affects scattered individual cells
Cells and organelles swell	Cells contract
Control of intracellular environment is lost, cells rupture and spill contents	Control of intracellular environment maintained, cytoplasm packaged as "apoptotic bodies"
	DOES NOT INDUCE INFLAMMATION
INDUCES INFLAMMATION	

Events Following Injury

The events following injury involve, in varying proportions, necrosis, inflammation, and repair. You can think of these processes as a temporal and morphologic continuum.

Necrosis is the death of Cells or tissue as a result of an Endogenous or Exogenous injury. Mild forms of injury may produce Sub-lethal cell injury without Necrosis, changes that are referred to as **Degeneration**.

Lethal and Sub-lethal cellular changes occur together in varying proportions.

Inflammation is the Vascular and Cellular response to necrosis or sub-lethal Cell injury and is the body's mechanism of limiting the spread of injury and removing Necrotic debris.

Repair refers to the body's attempt to replace dead cells, whether by **_Regeneration_** of the original tissue or **_Replacement_** by connective tissue.

Another type of Cellular death is referred to as **Apoptosis**, commonly described as Programmed Cell Death. Apoptotic Cell Death is not necessarily an indication of injury. It occurs, for example, during Embryogenesis when not all Cells generated are needed. It is also the mechanism of ridding the body of excess Lymphocytes following resolution of an inflammatory or immune event, of hormone-dependent cell death after the hormonal stimulus has been removed, and of tumor cell death.

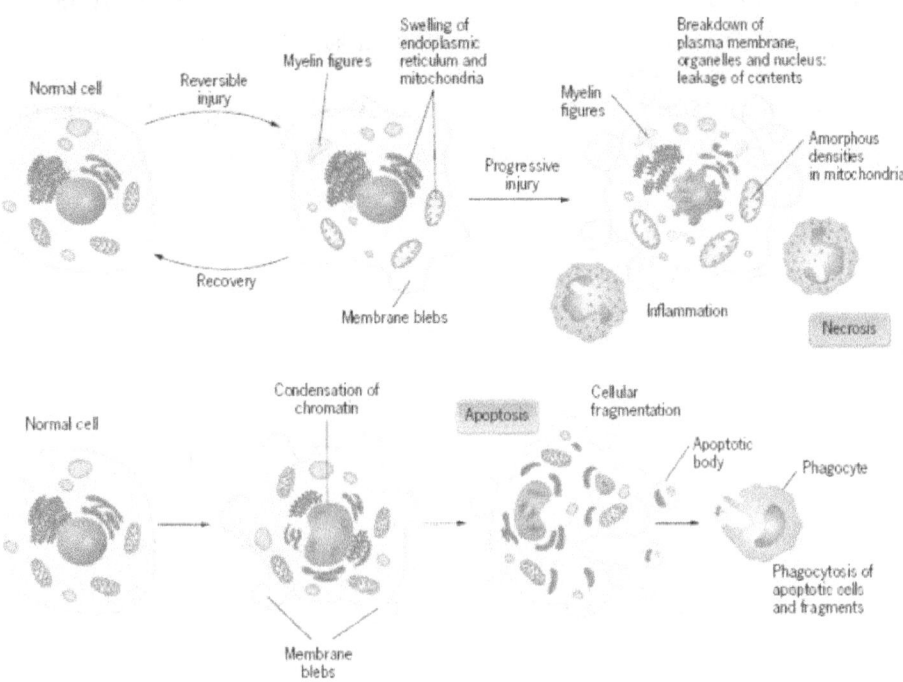

It may, however, also occur following injury from a variety of agents that might cause necrosis under other conditions.

Apoptosis is referred to as *Programmed* because it results from the Activation of specific Genes following appropriate stimuli.

In Tissue sections, it differs in appearance from necrosis in that the cell shrinks, the Nuclear Chromatin condenses into dense masses, Blebs form in the Cytoplasm, and the apoptotic cells are Phagocytosed by Macrophages or adjacent Parenchymal Cells. Importantly, Apoptosis does not elicit inflammation. Mainly for the latter reason, further discussion of cell death in this chapter concerns only Necrosis.

The relative intensities of Necrosis, Inflammation, and Repair depend on the magnitude of the injury, the duration of injury, and, to some extent, on the location within the body and the nature of the injury.

In general, Inflammation begins immediately after Cell Injury.

Repair is usually not well established until Necrosis ceases, although in very chronic injuries, all three processes are likely to occur together. When the Inflammation itself manifests at a certain level of intensity, it is considered a cause of Necrosis.

The body, in a sense, sacrifices some of its own tissue to isolate an injurious agent. This is just a glimpse into the AWESOME Natural abilities and Power of our Bodies. Which should go to ask WHY can't we Heal or Recover from certain dis-eases?

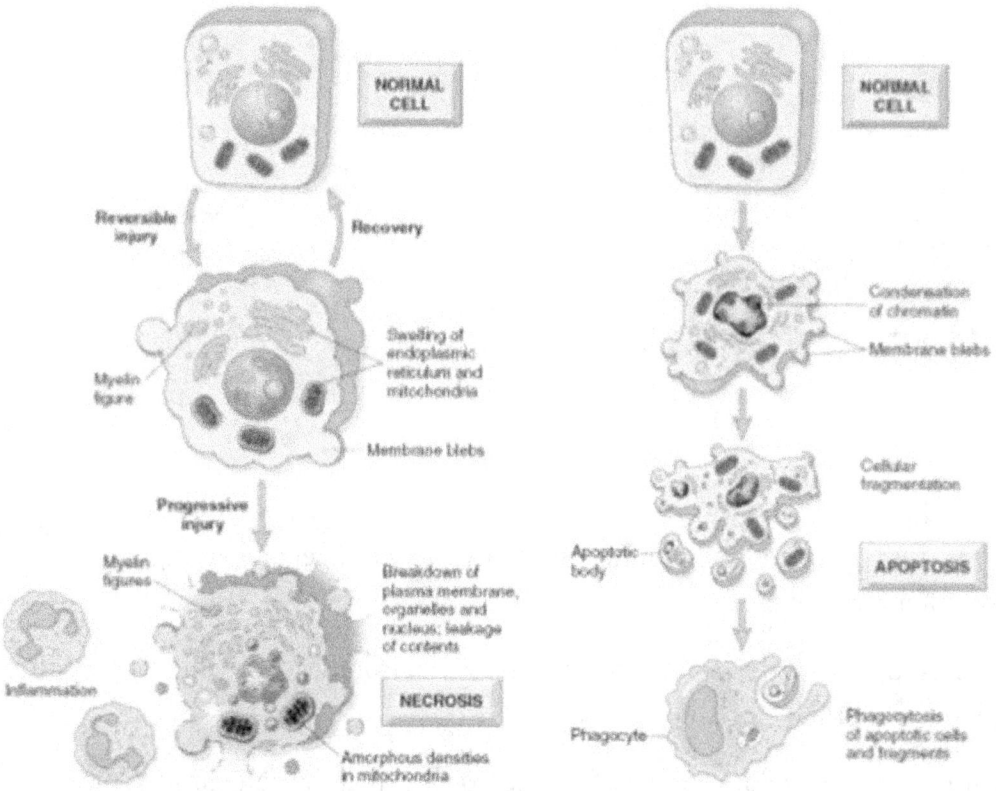

The critical difference between **Sub-lethal (reversible) Cell Injury** and Necrosis is whether the Cell can recover or is dead. Certain changes in the Nucleus, as seen in microscopic sections, indicate Cell Death.

Nuclear changes may include *Condensation* of the Nucleus (**Pyknosis**), *Fragmentation* of the Nucleus (**Karyorrhexis**), and *Lysis* or *Fading* of the Nucleus (**Karyolysis**).

These Nuclear changes take a number of hours to develop, so Cells may not show these changes Histologically even though they are dead.

For example, Heart Tissue in a person who dies within 12 hours of sustaining a Myocardial Infarct (heart attack) may not show the histologic changes of Necrosis. If the patient had lived, some of the Myocardial Cells would have developed the histologic changes of Necrosis, whereas others may have developed reversible changes and then recovered.

Reversible Cell Injury is characterized by Preservation of the nucleus and variable changes in the Cytoplasm such as Swelling or Condensation of the Cell, Nucleus, and/or Cytoplasmic Organelles. These histologic changes reflect Biochemical changes in the Cell.

There is no exact Biochemical End Point that determines Cell death….. but we do Know that a depletion in the Cell's Energy System (especially Adenosine Tri-Phosphate [ATP]) and alteration of Cell Membrane permeability are critical events leading to cell death.

Endogenous and Exogenous Causes of Tissue Injury

Endogenous	Exogenous
• Tissue necrosis	• Infections (bacterial, viral, or parasitic)
• Ischemia	
• Anoxia	• Trauma (blunt or penetrating)
• Immune reactions	• Physical agents
• Allergies	• Burns
• Autoimmune diseases	• Frostbite
• Hypersensitivity reactions	• Irradiation
	• Chemical agents
	• Acids
	• Bases
	• Environmental toxins
	• Foreign bodies

We are basically and simply several trillion of Cells – cooperating to create and maintain US! Which is WHY I decided to approach our Health and Fitness from this particular perspective.

By understanding HOW a Cell can or does die, we can KNOW how to keep it or Us ALIVE = Abundant Life!

There can be many different types of Cell Injuries that result, at least in part, from the generation of **Free Oxygen Radicals** that damage vital Cell structures such as the Membranes.

Free Radicals are essentially unstable Oxygen Molecules having only a single unpaired Electron in their outer orbit and are generated by the *Reduction* of Molecular Oxygen to Water.

They react with Proteins, Lipids, and Carbohydrates, releasing negative Energy that damages Membranes and corrupts the Cellular DNA that leads to a degenerative mutation that results in cancers, dis-eases and pre-mature death or Necrosis.

Acute Injury and Necrosis

Lack of Oxygen (**Anoxia**) or Reduced Oxygen (**Hypoxia**) is one of the most common causes of acute injury and necrosis. *I cover this aspect extensively in my book – 'OxyGen: The Breath Of Life in Atomic Form!', which is Volume 1 of my Science Of Life Series!*

Cells are vulnerable to Hypoxia in proportion to their Oxygen requirements; meaning that Metabolically Active Cells are selectively vulnerable.

Selective Vulnerability is well illustrated by cases of systemic Anoxia from such causes as Carbon Monoxide poisoning, blood loss, or suffocation. In these situations, Neurons in the Brain and the Kidneys' tubular Epithelial Cells are more vulnerable to Necrosis than are other types of Cells.

This science indicates that Brain death (mental and emotional instability) is one of the 1st manifested symptoms of Cellular Death.

Alzheimer's, dementia, depression, anxiety, mental retardation, loss of focus all represent symptoms of Cellular Injury leading to Necrosis, which is a strong indication of imminent pre-mature death of the whole Body.

Hypoxia and Anoxia both are effects that are direct results of using the Mouth for Respiration (Inhale or Exhale). Our Cells NEED Oxygen to function, produce Energy/ATP and maintain DNA.

Localized Hypoxia resulting from poor blood flow is called **Ischemia**. When severe, Ischemia leads to Necrosis of the Cells in the area of the compromised blood supply.

Because the Pulmonary Circuit is the 1st route of Blood – from the Heart to the Lungs to become Oxygenated, the 1st Organ to suffer ischemic Necrosis is the Heart.

An area of ischemic Necrosis is called an **Infarct**. Infarcts are most commonly caused by obstruction of Arteries. ***Atherosclerotic plaques that obstruct Coronary Arteries and lead to Myocardial Infarcts are responsible for a high percentage of all deaths***. Atherosclerotic obstruction also is important in producing Infarcts of the Brain, Legs, Kidneys, and other sites.

The Morphologic changes of Reversible Cell Injury and Necrosis form a continuum. If the injury is mild and functional changes following the injury go away in a few hours, the cells involved undergo Sub-lethal changes with an eventual return to their normal appearance.

If functional changes persist, it is likely that at least some Cells will undergo Necrosis; recovery then depends on regeneration, a process discussed later in the chapter. Study of biopsy specimens or tissues removed at autopsy allows the pathologist the opportunity to evaluate the extent of injury.

 Changes in reversibly damaged Cells are limited to the Cytoplasm; Necrotic Cells have both Cytoplasmic and Nuclear changes. Typically, the early change is Cytoplasmic swelling, producing enlarged Cells with pale Cytoplasm.

Later, the Cytoplasm may be shrunken and more densely Eosinophilic than normal. The development of Nuclear changes, manifested in the forms of—Pyknosis, Karyorrhexis, or Karyolysis—indicates a determined progression to Necrosis.

Thus, when Reversible Changes predominate, a Tissue is enlarged or when we see Swelling – meaning that we can save Self and Heal Self; but when Necrosis predominates, a Tissue is of normal size or shrunken – which indicates Life Ending.

Chronic Injury

Chronic injury may produce a decrease in Tissue size (**Atrophy**) or **Accumulation** of material within Cells or between Cells. Atrophy may be the result of a decrease in the *Size* of Cells, a decrease in the *Number* of Cells, or *Both*.

A gradual loss of Cells is the most common mechanism.

Chronic injuries associated with accumulation of substances are quite different from atrophy. Many times, Cells slowly accumulate their own Metabolic products or Exogenous materials, with a resultant decrease in cell function. The storage of these materials may even result in an enlarged cell, albeit one with *decreased function*. The types of chronic cell or tissue degeneration are classified according to the cause of the atrophy or type of material accumulated.

The CAUSE of Atrophy is predicated by either Trauma, HOW they are Breathing and/or WHAT they use for Food/Drink.

The TYPE of Material is based on HOW a person is Breathing (Mouth Inhalation allows for introduction of foreign elements) and HOW and WHAT they eat and drink.

Atrophy

Senile Atrophy is caused from the Aging Process when we Breathe, Drink and Eat wrong, causing Tissues to become smaller and decrease in functional capacity, *presumably* as a natural part of the aging process, but ACTUALLY caused by significant wear and tear on the Digestive System.

This wear and tear causes a severe impairment in the function and ability of Energy/Nutrient extraction and irreparable damage to our Immune System – which is WITHIN our Digestive System.

For an example, the brains of older people become smaller after 40, 50, 60 years of Breathing, Drinking and Eating wrong, which causes decreased memory and slowed thought processes. These provide some evidence of decreased Cellular Function, which leads to pre-mature Death.

Disuse Atrophy occurs when the Cells are unable to carry out their normal function. For example, when an arm or leg is placed in a cast, the muscle cells gradually become smaller and show a decreased ability to contract. Disuse atrophy may be reversible. Once the cast is removed and the limb is exercised, the atrophic muscle cells can regain their prior function and structure.

A SEDENTARY Lifestyle is becoming increasing related to Disuse Atrophy. Children are no longer as Active as they were 10-20 years ago, especially with the increased availability of electronically devices. So a Sedentary Lifestyle is beginning in Childhood instead of in old Age as it used to.

This means that Children aren't USING and Developing their normal and natural Muscular structure – Causing a DISUSE ATROPHY. Before a child reaches their early to mid 20's they have presented Serious medical issues with ASTHMA, Diabetes and Heart Problems as leading symptoms.

Today, OBESITY is risen to the point now that the Medical/Science field have to accept and classify CHILDHOOD DIABETES (primarily a result of Obesity) as a Dis-Ease and Epidemic!

However, if Muscle Cells are immobilized because of permanent loss of Nervous stimulation—for example, after the traumatic severance of a Nerve—they will stay atrophied. This type of atrophy is called **Denervation Atrophy.**

Pressure Atrophy results from steady pressure on Tissue, such as might be produced by the mass of an expanding tumor. Bedsores are another common example. They occur in chronically bedridden patients because of continued external pressure on the skin. Walking, Standing, Sitting, Laying, Running and Moving run over 10, 20, 30 years creates Pressure Atrophy, usually manifesting in the Lumbar region of the Back.

Endocrine Atrophy results from decreased Hormonal stimulation. Certain Organs are maintained in a functional state by the action of Hormones on them. Insufficient Hormonal stimulation results in Atrophy in that Organ. For an example, the decrease in Estrogen and Progesterone at the time of Menopause results in Atrophy of the Breasts and the Uterus.

The Endocrine System is Food Sensitive, and the Cells NEED Oxygen and Glucose to maintain and reproduce properly. HOW we Breathe and WHAT and HOW we eat and drink

Accumulations

Various substances can accumulate within cells. Accumulation of lipid within cells is called **Fatty Change** or Fatty Metamorphosis. Fatty Change should be distinguished from **Adiposity**. In Adiposity, there is an increased storage of Fat in Fat Cells; in Fatty change, Fat droplets appear as an abnormality in Parenchymal Cells.

Fatty change may be either *acute* or *chronic* and characteristically occurs in Cells that are involved in Fat metabolism, especially the Liver. The Liver takes in Lipid in the form of Triglycerides (from dietary absorption/extraction) and Free Fatty Acids (from Adipose Tissue stores or absorption). The Liver then metabolizes these Triglycerides and Free Fatty Acids into Lipoprotein, a much more soluble form of Lipid that can be exported and transferred for use by other Tissues.

Droplets of Triglyceride may form in Hepatocytes because of decreased production of Lipoprotein or increased uptake of Lipid from the Blood. The Causes of Fatty Liver include conditions that induce mobilization of more Fat than the Liver can handle, such as diabetes mellitus; excess food intake; eating the wrong foods; chemical injury, as in alcoholism or Carbon Tetrachloride poisoning; and acute starvation, where there is depletion of the proteins needed to form Lipoproteins.

In diabetes mellitus, there is decreased uptake of Fat in Adipose Tissue and increased accumulation in the Liver.

In chronic alcoholism, the Liver may become more than twice its normal size as a result of the accumulation of Fat in the form of Hepatocytes. *Alcoholism is the most common cause of clinically significant fatty liver in affluent societies.*

Effects of Injury

Causes
Physical injury
Chemical injury
Infection
Anoxia/ischemia
Antigen–antibody reactions
Metabolic abnormalities
Radiation
Lesions
Reversible cell changes
Necrosis
Atrophy
Accumulations
Manifestations
Loss of cell function related to site involved

Inflammation

Inflammation is the naturally occurring protective response that the body mounts in response to injury. This term reflects the observation that an inflamed lesion is like fire: red, hot, and painful. Wherein Necrosis reflects the destructive effects of injury to Cells, Inflammation is a process by which Fluid, Chemicals, and Cells are brought to an injured area to **Limit** the extent of Injury, **Remove** Necrotic debris, and **Prepare** for the healing process.

Inflammation involves very complex Chemical and, to a lesser extent, Neural mechanisms that serve to turn the "***fire fighters***" on quickly and mobilize more reserves, but also to turn the process off so that these Cellular and Chemical responses do not destroy any more normal Tissue than is necessary to control the spread of injury.

Inflammation: Body's response to injury

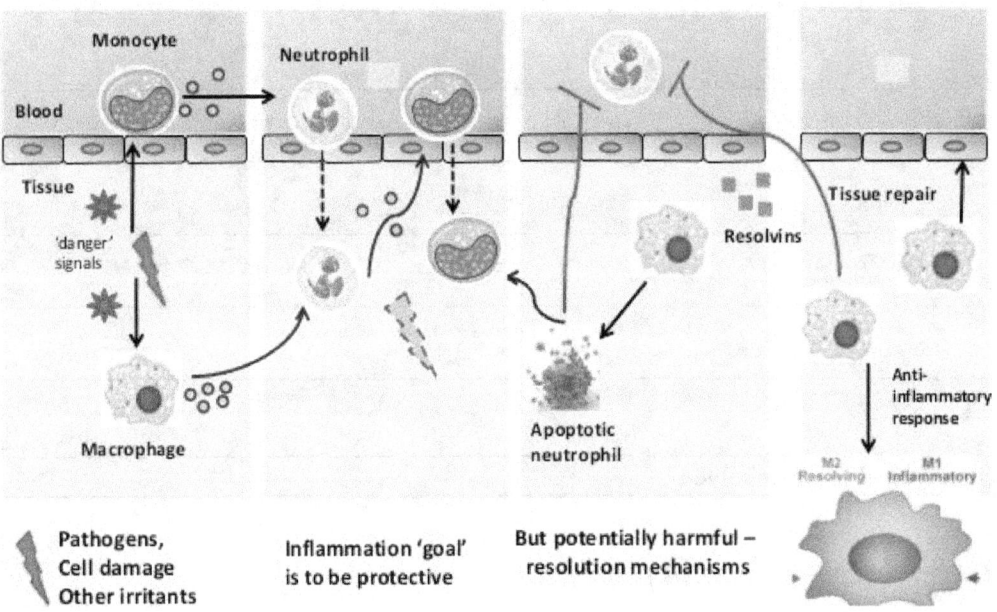

The nature of the Inflammatory response, the degree and duration vary depending on the **cause** and **time** course of the injury. Although inflammation is described as a protective response, it also has damaging effects.

The potential for drugs to modify the inflammatory response has stimulated continued research to unravel its complex biochemical control mechanisms. Because these drugs or biochemical mechanisms are man-made, they don't present the best response to an Inflammatory situation.

Attempting to unnaturally Modify a Natural response significantly interferes with the natural Healing process – which may be the root cause in the increase and severity of dis-eases and the mortality rates.

This makes our choices of food and drink even more important and necessary to successfully Build and Maintain Supreme Health and Fitness!

Acute Inflammation

Acute Inflammation consists of tightly coordinated Vascular and Cellular responses to injury. The Vascular response results in ***increased*** Blood flow to the injured area and ***increased*** Vascular permeability so that Water, Electrolytes, and Serum Proteins ***leak*** into the tissue spaces.

The Cellular response refers to the movement of Leukocytes, predominantly Neutrophils and Monocytes, from the Blood into the Tissue.

These events produce the **Cardinal Signs of Inflammation**: redness, swelling, heat, pain, and loss of function. The increased Blood flow in ***dilated*** vessels is called **Hyperemia** and causes redness. The leakage of fluid into the Tissue is called **Edema** and causes swelling. The increased Blood in the area causes **Heat**. **Pain** results from the pressure of the swelling and the action of Kinins on nerve endings. **Loss of Function** results from the attempt to protect the painful, swollen lesion from further injury.

The effects of inflammation are to destroy or limit the spread of the causative agent and to clean up the debris in preparation for repair. In simple injuries, such as a burn, a cut, or a chemical injury where the chemical has been diluted away, the causative agent is no longer a threat and the inflammatory reaction is proportional to the amount of tissue damage. Tissue damage itself incites a mild inflammatory reaction, enough to bring Leukocytes to digest and remove the debris from the dead cells and increase Lymph flow to carry away fluid from the lesion.

Acute Inflammation

Causes
All types of acute injuries (necrosis)
Pyogenic infections
Hypersensitivities
Lesions
Hyperemia
Exudate
Neutrophils and macrophages
Manifestations
Redness
Heat
Swelling
Pain
Loss of function
Fever
Leukocytosis
Chronic Inflammation

Chronic means persistent for a long time. In that sense, chronic inflammation may result from acute inflammation that persists because the cause is not completely eliminated, or it may be associated with a cause that never was acute but is continuing at a low level for a long time.

The term *chronic inflammation* is also used as a label for the histologic picture typically associated with prolonged inflammation.

Natural Healing, Repair & Regeneration

The body's two basic methods of repair following tissue destruction are **Regeneration** and **Fibrous Connective Tissue Repair** (scarring or fibrosis). Regeneration is replacement of the destroyed Tissue by Cells *similar* to those previously present—that is, the Parenchymal Cells of the Organ are *reconstituted*.

Time sequences of necrosis (N), inflammation (I), and repair (R).

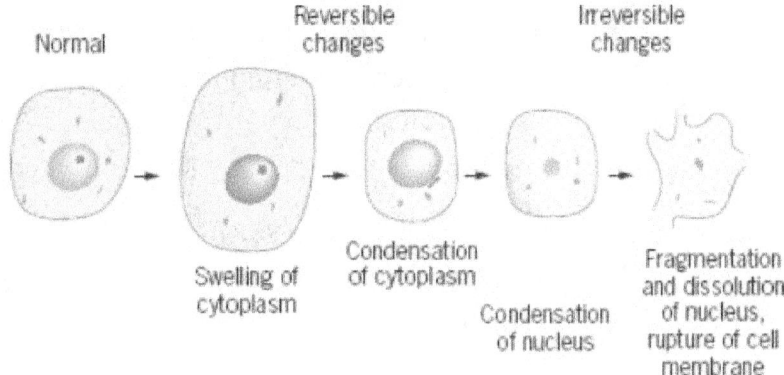

For an example, the Epidermal surface of a cut is replaced by Epidermis, fractured Bone is united by Bone, and scattered dead Liver Cells are replaced by new Liver Cells.

This is the Natural Ability of our Bodies – WITHOUT Us doing anything medically to assist. Imagine that we Breathed, Drank and Ate according to our Nature and Anatomical function = TOTAL BODY HEALING, REPAIR & REGENERATION!

We would create an atmosphere IN self of constant and consistent Health and Wellness = Abundant Life!

In the Fibrous Connective Tissue Repair, the Tissue previously present is replaced by Fibrous Tissue (scar). For an example, the Dermal edges of a cut are *united* by Scar, a Bone fracture that is not properly united is *healed* by Scar Tissue, and extensively damaged Liver may be *replaced* by Fibrous Tissue.

Many tissue injuries *heal* in part by Regeneration and in part by Fibrosis.

Regeneration is the most desirable form of Repair because **normal function** is Restored. Regeneration of Functional Tissue is particularly important when there has been widespread damage to a vital organ.

As a prerequisite to regeneration, cells next to those that have died must be able to multiply and this is mainly determined by whether we are Breathing properly, Hydrated and Eating to Live. If we are performing each of these Life Functions properly, the surrounding Cells will be Healthy enough to Stop the Injury and successfully Repair and Regenerate the injured Cell.

Some Cells, such as Neurons and Cardiac Muscle Fibers, do not undergo Cell division in adults; therefore, these Cells cannot regenerate after injuries. In contrast, tissues that are continuously replacing their cells under normal circumstances, such as the cells of the epidermis, gastrointestinal tract, or bone, have a great capacity for regeneration.

*It must be noted that the research and results on the lack of Regeneration in the Neurons and Cardiac Muscle in Adults is based mainly on adults that performed one or more of the 3 Life Functions incorrectly.

By the age of 5, 95% of the children have begun to breathe wrong = Mouth and Chest Breathing, which means that by adulthood the average persons Cardiac Muscle is already injured from Lack of Oxygen or Oxygen deficiency.

This would significantly impair Regeneration, making it almost virtually impossible – leading to NON-REGENERATION = PRE- MATURE DEATH!

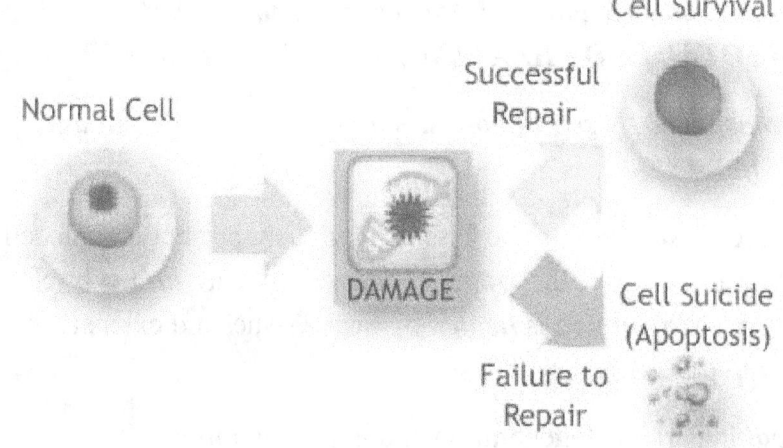

The Epidermis and Intestinal Mucosa can repair defects up to several centimeters in diameter through the process of Regeneration. Bone Marrow can replace itself even when only a few Cells survive an injury. Its tremendous capacity to Regenerate from only a few Cells is exploited therapeutically in Bone Marrow transplants. The diseased bone marrow is first ablated by toxic drugs, and then a few cells from a donor are introduced and completely reconstitute functional bone marrow.

Most of the Tissues of the Body normally undergo Cell Replacement at a slow rate and are intermediate in their ability to Regenerate.

Regeneration can usually occur in Parenchymal Organs if the architectural framework is not destroyed. Complex structures composed of Interrelating Tissue types, such as the gas-exchanging membranes of the Lung and Renal Glomeruli, do not Regenerate.

The above naturally occurring scientific and chemical reactions of Self-Healing, Repair and Regeneration can be Increased and Accelerated by proper performing of our 3 Life Functions.

We would be able to successfully Enjoy Abundant Life!

Fibrous Connective Tissue Repair (Scarring or Fibrosis)

Fibrosis can occur in any Tissue and produces the same result regardless of site—namely, the formation of a dense, tough mass of Collagen called a **Scar**. Unlike Regeneration, Replacement by Fibrous Tissue does not restore the original function. The purpose of Fibrosis is to provide a strong bridge across the damaged area.

The process of Fibrous repair is also called **Organization** and consists of a Granulation Tissue stage and a Scar Formation stage. **Granulation Tissue** consists of Capillaries and Fibroblasts. Repair is initiated by the ingrowth of new Capillaries and Fibroblasts into the injured area. The Capillaries bring blood to provide the nutrition for the Repair process. *Capillaries also carry away liquid remains of dead tissue and particulate material removed by macrophages*.

This removal process is called **Resolution**. The f\Fibroblasts proliferate rapidly and then initiate the stage of Scar Formation by laying down Collagen.

Initially, there are small amounts of loose Collagen within the mass of Capillaries and Fibroblasts. With time, more Collagen is formed and the number of Capillaries and Fibroblasts decreases. The final stage, which takes weeks to months, involves shrinking and condensation of the Fibrous scar.

Wound Repair

The process of repairing wounds is artificially separated into repair by a Primary Union and Secondary Union, depending on whether the wound edges are placed together or left separated. The best example of repair by primary union is that which follows a clean surgical incision of the skin in which there is minimal tissue damage and the edges of the wound are closely approximated by tape or sutures.

In this example, the narrow space between the two wound edges fills with a small amount of serum, which quickly dries and clots, forming a scab. Within 1 to 2 days, the narrow zone of Acute Inflammation at the wound edges has lessened and new Capillaries begin to bridge the gap across the defect. By this time, the Epithelium has already grown across the surface of the gap.

Within a few more days, Fibroblasts grow across the sub-epithelial portions of the wound and begin to deposit Collagen, which eventually contracts, pulling the wound edges together and giving them Strength. Although this incision may appear well healed by about 2 weeks, it may take a month or more for the strength of the scar tissue to approximate that of the original tissue.

This is just an example at the Amazing naturally occurring Healing and Regeneration abilities of our Bodies. With just a little concentrated effort of ensuring that we are Breathing properly, being adequately Hydrated and Eating to Live, we can Immediately Improve the Quality of our Lives while simultaneously Extending our Life-Span.

This represents the Core Belief of Supreme Health and Fitness.

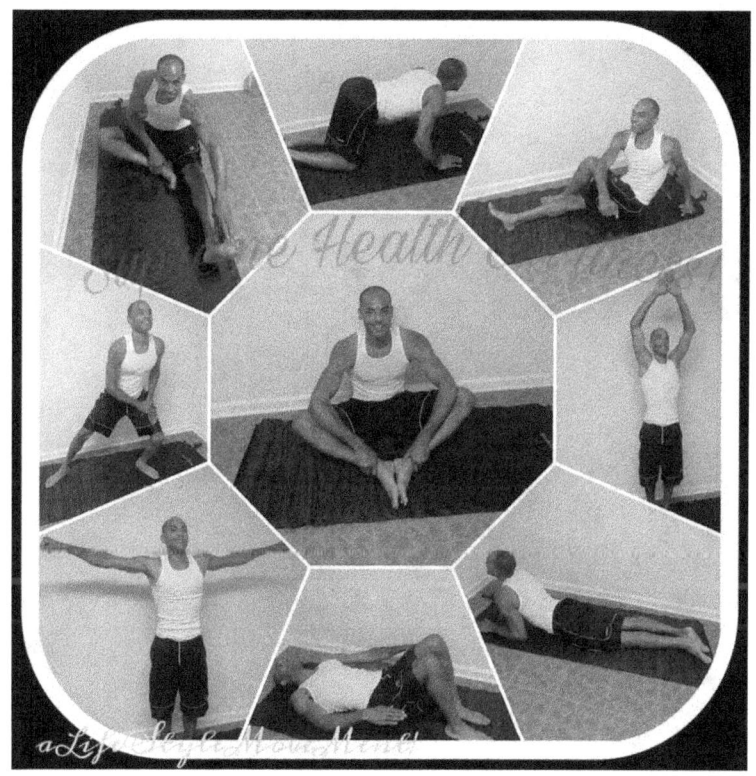

The 5 Fitness Components

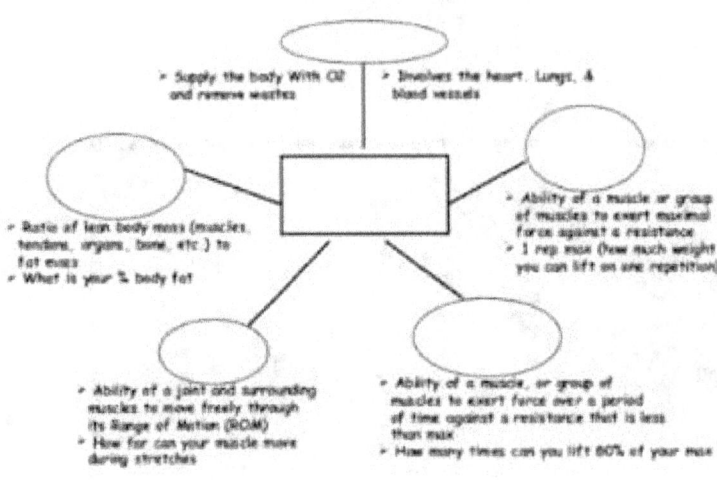

> Supply the body With O2 and remove wastes

> Involves the heart, Lungs, & blood vessels

> Ability of a muscle or group of muscles to exert maximal force against a resistance
> 1 rep max (how much weight you can lift on one repetition)

> Ratio of lean body mass (muscles, tendons, organs, bone, etc.) to fat mass
> What is your % body fat

> Ability of a joint and surrounding muscles to move freely through its Range of Motion (ROM)
> How far can your muscle move during stretches

> Ability of a muscle, or group of muscles to exert force over a period of time against a resistance that is less than max
> How many times can you lift 80% of your max

Chapter 6 ...

Physical Activity & Health

*****

There are many studies covering a range of issues where researchers have specifically focused on Exercise as well as on the more broadly defined concept of Physical Activity. Exercise is a form of physical activity that is planned, structured, repetitive, and performed with the goal of improving health or fitness.

So, although all exercise is physical activity, not all physical activity is exercise.

Studies have examined the role of physical activity in many groups—men and women, children, teens, adults, older adults, people with disabilities, and women during pregnancy and the postpartum period.

These studies have focused on the role that physical activity plays in many health outcomes, including:

- premature (early) death;

- dis-eases such as coronary heart disease, stroke, some cancers, type 2 diabetes, osteoporosis, and depression;

- risk factors for dis-ease, such as high blood pressure and high blood cholesterol;

- physical fitness, such as aerobic capacity, and muscle strength and endurance;

- functional capacity (the ability to engage in activities needed for daily living);

- mental health, such as depression and cognitive function; and

- injuries or sudden heart attacks.

These studies have also prompted serious questions regarding what type and how much physical activity is needed for various health benefits.

To answer this question, investigators have studied three main kinds of physical activity: aerobic, muscle strengthening, and bone strengthening, addressed in later chapters.

Fitness

- A. Being active improves health: 30 minutes of accumulated physical activity on most days of the week
- B. Being "fit" goes beyond health and requires a comprehensive exercise program that includes the following components
- 1) Cardiorespiratory endurance
- 2) Muscular strength and endurance
- 3) Flexibility
- 4) Body composition
- 5) Balance

Health Benefits of Physical Activity

There are several studies that clearly demonstrate that participating in regular physical activity provides many health benefits. Many conditions affected by physical activity occur with increasing age, such as heart disease and cancer. Reducing risk of these conditions may require years of participation in regular physical activity.

However, other benefits, such as increased **Cardiorespiratory Fitness**, increased muscular strength, and decreased depressive symptoms and blood pressure, require only a few weeks or months of participation in physical activity, *which means that by Beginning Tomorrow = Immediate Positive Health results.*

Components of Fitness

- 1) Cardiorespiratory endurance
  - The ability to perform large muscle movements over a sustained period
- 2a) Muscular strength
  - The max force that a muscle can produce against a resistance in a single maximal effort.
- 2b) Endurance
  - The capacity of a muscle to exert force repeatedly against a resistance

Movement is the Foundation of LIFE, starting with the Rotation of the ATOM.

The health benefits of physical activity are wide-ranging and seen in children and adolescents, young and middle-aged adults, older adults, women and men, people of different races and ethnicities, and people with disabilities and chronic conditions.

The health benefits of physical activity are generally independent of body weight. Adults of all sizes and shapes gain health and fitness benefits by being habitually physically active. The benefits of physical activity also outweigh the risk of injury and sudden heart attacks, two concerns that prevent many people from becoming physically active.

Components of Fitness

- 3) Flexibility
  - The range of motion around a joint
- 4) Body composition
  - The make-up of the body in terms of the relative percentage of fat free mass and body fat
- 5) Balance
  - The ability to maintain the body's position over it's base of support.

Health and Avoidance of Disease

What does being healthy mean? For some it is the simple avoidance of disease, but it is also a lot more than that.

Health has been defined as a human condition possessing social, psychological, and physical dimensions.

Positive health is associated with a capacity to enjoy life and withstand challenges.

Negative health is associated with morbidity (incidence of disease) and premature mortality.

The Highest Quality of life includes Mental alertness and curiosity, Positive emotional feelings, meaningful relationships with others, awareness and involvement in societal strivings, recognition of the broader forces of Life, and the physical capacity to accomplish personal goals with vigor.

These aspects of positive health are interrelated and a high level of accomplishment in one area *enhances* the other areas, and, conversely, a low level of function in any area *restricts* the accomplishments possible in other areas.

Although physical activity plays a major role in the physical dimension, it also *contributes* to learning, relationships, and a sense of human limitations within the broader perspective.

An optimal Quality of Life requires individuals to strive, grow, and develop. To Successfully Build and Maintain YOUR own Supreme Health and Fitness requires proper Physical Activity/Motion.

What are the risks or challenges to YOUR Health and Well-being?

Children and Adolescents

Strong evidence

- Improved cardiorespiratory and muscular fitness
- Improved bone health
- Improved cardiovascular and metabolic health biomarkers
- Favorable body composition

Moderate evidence

- Reduced symptoms of depression

Adults and Older Adults

Strong evidence

- Lower risk of early death
- Lower risk of coronary heart disease
- Lower risk of stroke
- Lower risk of high blood pressure
- Lower risk of adverse blood lipid profile
- Lower risk of type 2 diabetes
- Lower risk of metabolic syndrome
- Lower risk of colon cancer
- Lower risk of breast cancer
- Prevention of weight gain
- Weight loss, particularly when combined with reduced calorie intake
- Improved cardiorespiratory and muscular fitness
- Prevention of falls
- Reduced depression
- Better cognitive function (for older adults)

Moderate to strong evidence

- Better functional health (for older adults)
- Reduced abdominal obesity

Moderate evidence

- Lower risk of hip fracture
- Lower risk of lung cancer
- Lower risk of endometrial cancer
- Weight maintenance after weight loss
- Increased bone density
- Improved sleep quality

Reduced Risk of Premature Death

There is Strong scientific evidence that shows that physical activity reduces the risk of pre-mature death (dying earlier than the average age-at-death for a specific population group) from the *leading causes* of death, such as heart disease and some cancers, as well as from other causes of death.

This effect is remarkable in two ways:

■ *First*, only a few lifestyle choices have as large an effect on mortality as physical activity. It has been estimated that people who are *physically active for approximately 7 hours a week have a 40% lower risk of dying early* than those who are active for less than 30 minutes a week.

■ *Second*, it is not necessary to do high amounts of physical activity or vigorous-intensity activity to reduce the risk of premature death. Studies show substantially lower risk when people do *150 minutes of at least moderate-intensity aerobic physical activity a week.*

Cardiorespiratory Health

The *benefits* of physical activity on Cardiorespiratory health are some of the most extensively documented of all the health benefits. Cardiorespiratory health simply involves the health of the Heart, Lungs, and Blood Vessels.

The Cardio-Vascular System is our Engine. When our Heart STOPS beating and pumping Oxygenated Blood = we are DEAD.

In fact, the one difference between a Life and Death is the ability to Breathe!

Heart dis-eases and stroke are two of the leading causes of death in the United States.

Risk factors that *increase* the likelihood of Cardiovascular dis-eases include smoking, high blood pressure (called Hypertension), type 2 diabetes, and high levels of certain blood lipids (such as Low-Density Lipoprotein, or LDL, Cholesterol).

Low Cardiorespiratory fitness is also a *risk factor* for heart disease.

People who do moderate- or vigorous-intensity aerobic physical activity have a *significantly lower* risk of Cardiovascular disease than do inactive people.

Regularly active adults have *lower* rates of heart disease and stroke, *lower* Blood Pressure, *better* Blood Lipid profiles, and *better* over-all fitness.

Significant *reductions* in risk of Cardiovascular dis-ease are observed at activity levels equivalent to *150 minutes a week of moderate-intensity physical activity*.

Even *greater benefits are seen with 200 minutes* (3 hours and 20 minutes) a week. The evidence is strong that *greater* amounts of physical activity result in even further *reductions* in the risk of Cardiovascular dis-ease.

Everyone can gain the Cardiovascular health benefits of physical activity.

The amount of physical activity that provides favorable cardiorespiratory health and fitness outcomes is similar for adults of various ages, including older people, as well as for adults of various races and ethnicities. Aerobic exercise also improves Cardiorespiratory fitness in individuals with some disabilities, including people who have lost the use of one or both legs and those with multiple sclerosis, stroke, spinal cord injury, and cognitive disabilities.

Moderate-intensity physical activity is safe for generally healthy women during pregnancy. It *increases* Cardiorespiratory fitness without increasing the risk of early pregnancy loss, preterm delivery, or low birth weight.

Physical activity during the postpartum period also improves cardiorespiratory fitness.

The First Law of Thermodynamics
(i.e., energy conservation)

$$\Delta E = E_{in} - E_{out}$$

Change in fat mass = Energy consumed − Energy expended

Metabolic Health

Regular physical activity **strongly reduces** the risk of developing type 2 diabetes as well as the Metabolic Syndrome. The Metabolic Syndrome is a condition in which people have some **combination** of high blood pressure, a large waistline (abdominal obesity), an adverse blood lipid profile (low levels of high-density lipoprotein [HDL] cholesterol, raised triglycerides), and impaired Glucose tolerance.

People who regularly engage in at least **moderate-intensity** Aerobic activity have a **significantly lower risk** of developing type 2 diabetes than do inactive people. Although some experts debate the usefulness of defining the metabolic syndrome, good evidence exists that physical activity reduces the risk of having this condition, as defined in various ways.

Lower rates of these conditions are seen with *120 to 150 minutes* (2 hours to 2 hours and 30 minutes) a week of at least moderate-intensity Aerobic activity. As with cardiovascular health, additional levels of physical activity lower the risk even further. In addition, physical activity helps control blood glucose levels in persons who already have type 2 diabetes.

Physical Activity Guidelines

Given the large number of benefits derived from participation in physical activity, it should be no surprise that professional societies such as the American College of Sports Medicine (ACSM), the American Heart Association (AHA), and various governmental agencies (e.g., Centers for Disease Control and Prevention [CDC]) have developed physical activity guidelines for the general public.

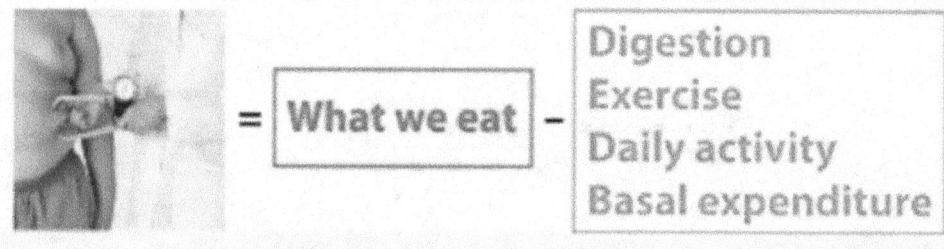

Vigorous Exercise, Fitness, and Health

In the early and mid-1970s, three major organizations published guidelines or recommendations for improving fitness and health:

1. In 1972, the AHA published *Exercise Testing and Training of Apparently Healthy Individuals: A Handbook for Physicians* (5). The exercise prescription was to begin at 75% HRmax for 15 to 20 min, 3 days $\cdot$ wk^{-1}.

2. In 1973, the YMCA published it first edition of *The Y's Way to Physical Fitness* (16). The exercise prescription was to exercise at 80% VO$_2$max for 40 to 45 min, 3 days $\cdot$ wk^{-1}.

3. In 1975, ACSM published the first edition of *ACSM's Guidelines for Exercise Testing and Prescription* (1). The exercise prescription was to exercise at ~70% to 90% O$_2$max for 20 to 45 min, 3 to 5 days $\cdot$ wk^{-1}.

In each case the focus was on higher-intensity exercise, with both CRF and health outcomes being important.

Volume of Physical Activity and Health Outcomes

In 1978, ACSM published its first position stand: "The Recommended Quantity and Quality of Exercise for Developing and Maintaining Fitness in Healthy Adults."

The focus was on improving CRF as well as achieving health outcomes.

The emphasis was again on higher-intensity exercise to achieve these goals.

However, in that same year, a now classic study on Harvard alumni by Paffenbarger, Wing, and Hyde showed a 36% lower risk of developing a heart attack in those who accumulated 2,000 kilocalories or more of leisure-time physical activity per week (that did not have to be done at a high intensity).

This study and many that followed shifted the focus to three variables associated with physical activity guidelines:

• Activity volume (e.g., kilocalories expended) rather than intensity

• Health outcomes (e.g., reduced risk of heart attack) rather than CRF

• Leisure activity rather than structured exercise programs

Throughout the 1980s there was a growing body of research showing a strong relationship between regular participation in physical activity and a lower risk of chronic disease. It became clear that we needed to rethink our understanding of how physical activity and exercise were linked to a reduced risk of chronic disease. Dr. William Haskell took a leadership role in helping us to understand the potential links among physical activity, fitness, and health (in below figure) shows the following:

• In our earliest understanding, we thought that physical activity improved fitness, which, in turn, was linked to improved health outcomes (number 1).

• However, it was just as likely that physical activity could improve health and fitness separately and by different mechanisms (number 2).

1. Physical activity → Fitness → Health

2. Physical activity → Fitness → Health

3. Physical activity → Fitness; Physical activity → Health

4. Physical activity → Health; Physical activity → Fitness

• Lastly, *some* physical activity programs could improve fitness and not health outcomes, and vice versa (numbers 3 and 4).

These distinctions helped shape our understanding of how physical activity is connected to fitness and health outcomes, that is, physical activity could achieve health outcomes independent of fitness.

Physical Activity and Obesity

The United States and many other industrialized countries have seen an incredible increase in the prevalence of overweight and obesity over the last 20 years. In the United States, *32.3% of men* and *35.5% of women* are OBESE, with *combined* overweight and obesity prevalence being *68% and 72.3%*, respectively.

The increase in obesity during the 1990s prompted the Institute of Medicine (IOM) to evaluate the research on how much physical activity was needed to prevent weight gain. The IOM recommended 60 minutes of *moderate-intensity* activity to prevent weight gain and achieve the full health benefits of physical activity, twice the amount that ACSM and the CDC recommended for reducing the risk of chronic diseases.

This was supported by recommendations from the International Association for the Study of Obesity (IASO) to do 45 to 60 min of physical activity to prevent weight gain and the International Obesity Task Force (IOTF) recommendation of *60 to 90 minutes of activity* to prevent weight regain in those who have lost a great deal of weight.

In 2005, the *Dietary Guidelines for Americans* endorsed the ACSM and CDC recommendation of 30 min of physical activity to reduce the risk of chronic diseases, the IOM recommendation of 60 min to prevent weight gain, and the IOTF recommendation of 60 to 90 min to sustain weight loss.

Factors Affecting Health and Disease

The *five leading causes of death* in the United States in 2007 were Cardiovascular diseases (CVD) (31.0%), Cancers (23.2%), chronic lower-respiratory diseases (5.3%), accidents (5.1%), and Alzheimer's disease (3.1%). Although infectious diseases are not in the top five, we are warned each year to make sure that our flu shots and other vaccinations are up to date in order to prevent a problem from occurring.

ALL of the top five leading causes of death are Chronic Degenerative dis-eases whose onset can be delayed or prevented.

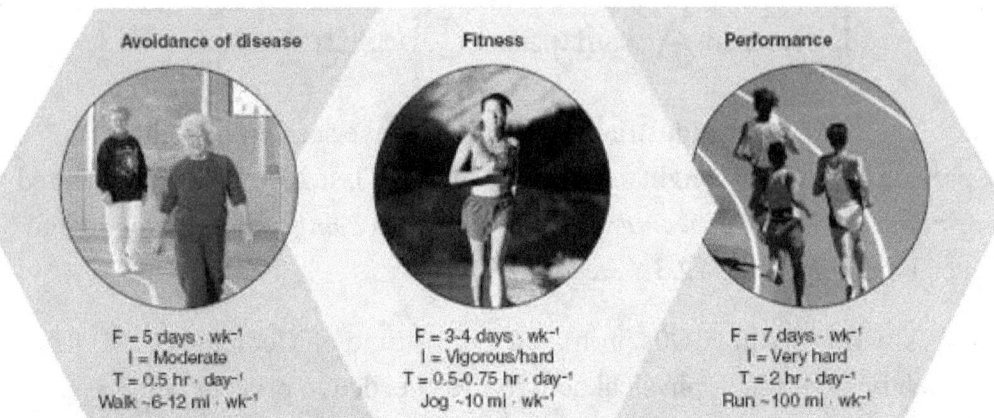

Risk factors associated with chronic diseases can be divided into three categories:

1. Inherited or Biological Factors

These factors include the following:

• *Age*—older adults have more chronic diseases than younger people.

• *Gender*—men develop CVD at an earlier age than women, but women experience more strokes than men.

• *Race*—African Americans develop about 30% more heart disease than non-Hispanic white Americans.

• *Susceptibility to disease*—several diseases have a genetic component that increases the potential for having them.

People can achieve health and fitness goals up to their genetic potential, but it is not possible to establish the relative portion of a person's health that is determined by heredity.

Although heredity does influences physical activity, fitness, and health, most people can lead healthy or unhealthy lives regardless of their genetic makeup because true Health and Fitness requires proper Respiration, Hydration and Energy/Nutrition

Thus, genetic background neither dooms a person to poor health nor guarantees good health.

2. Environment

We are born not only with fixed genetic potentials but also into environments that affect our development. An environment includes physical factors (e.g., climate, water, altitude, pollution), socioeconomic factors (e.g., income, housing, education, workplace characteristics), and family (e.g., parental values, divorce, extended family, friends) that affect our opportunities to be active, level of fitness, and health status.

Some elements, such as our nutrition or the air we breathe and water we drink, affect us directly. Other elements, such as the values and behaviors of people we admire, influence our lifestyles indirectly.

We can control certain aspects of our environments; for instance, we choose many of the mental and physical activities we undertake. However, our past and current environments affect us in various ways. For example, some children have inadequate food because of their environment and cannot think about other aspects of health until that basic need is fulfilled.

3. Behaviors

We have discussed the leading causes of death, but what are the *actual causes* of death? That smoking is at the top of the list should be no surprise given its connection to both lung cancer and CVD. In fact, it is **the number one actual cause of death**, accounting for **18% of all deaths**. The existence of smoking-cessation programs and laws to restrict areas in which one can smoke speak to the seriousness with which our society takes that risk to health.

The **number two actual cause of death is poor diet and physical inactivity** (15.2%), with alcohol consumption coming in at number three (3.5%).

If we eliminate Smoking, Poor dietary choices and Increase Physical Activity we will have Successfully prevented Self from succumbing to the 2 major forms of pre-mature death!

The emphasis on healthy eating at work and school and the creation of new parks and bike trails to enhance opportunities to be physically active are examples of responses to these actual causes of death.

Healthy eating and physical activity affect a large number of factors that influence health and disease.

Physical activity also *improves* Metabolic health in our youth. There are several studies that have found this positive effect when young people participate in at *least 3 days* of vigorous aerobic activity a week.

More physical activity is associated with improved metabolic health, but research has yet to determine the exact amount of improvement.

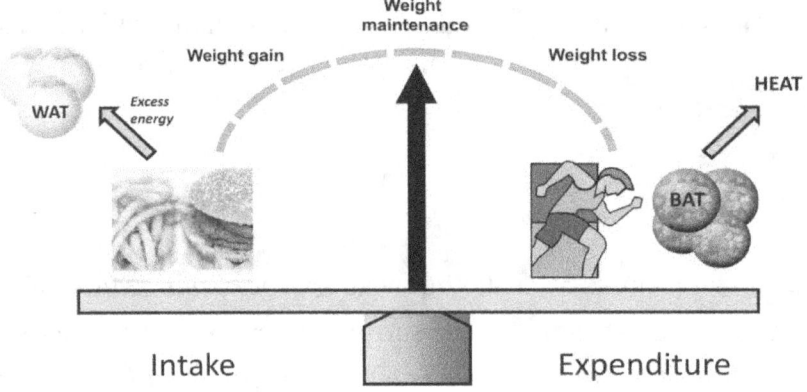

Weight and Energy Balance

Overweight and Obesity occur when *fewer* calories are *expended*, including Calories burned through physical activity, than are *taken in* through food and beverages.

Physical activity and *caloric intake* both must be considered when trying to control body weight. Because of this role in Energy Balance, *physical activity is a critical factor* in determining whether a person can maintain a healthy body weight, lose excess body weight, or maintain successful weight loss.

Health and Wellness is intensely Personal and Individualistic. Because of Genetics and other pre-dispositions and existing conditions people vary a great deal in how much physical activity they need to achieve and maintain a healthy weight. Some need more physical activity than others to maintain a healthy body weight, to lose weight, or to keep weight off once it has been lost.

Strong scientific evidence shows that physical activity helps people maintain a stable weight over time. However, the optimal amount of physical activity needed to maintain weight is unclear because it has to be based on the specific individuals health needs.

People vary greatly in how much physical activity results in weight stability. Many people need more than the equivalent of 150 minutes of moderate-intensity activity a week to maintain their weight.

Over short periods of time, such as a year, research shows that it is possible to achieve weight stability by doing the equivalent of 150 to 300 minutes (5 hours) a week of moderate-intensity walking at about a 4-mile-an-hour pace.

Muscle-strengthening activities may help promote weight maintenance, although not to the significant degree as Aerobic activity.

People who want to lose a substantial (more than 5% of body weight) amount of weight and people who are trying to keep a significant amount of weight off once it has been lost need a high amount of physical activity, unless they also reduce their caloric intake. Many people need to do more than 300 minutes of moderate-intensity activity a week to meet weight–control goals.

Regular physical activity also helps control the percentage of Body Fat in children and adolescents, which significantly decreases the possibility of being over-weight or obese and suffering from the associated dis-eases, mainly childhood diabetes.

Exercise training studies with overweight and obese youth have shown that they can *reduce* their body fat by participating in physical activity that is at least of ***moderate-intensity for 3 to 5 days a week,*** at ***30 to 60 minutes each time.***

Musculoskeletal Health

Bones, Muscles, and Joints support the Body and help it Move and maintain continual Motion. Healthy Bones, Joints, and Muscles are *critical* to the ability to do daily activities *without* physical limitations.

Preserving Bone, Joint, and Muscle health is *essential* with increasing age. Studies show that the frequent decline in Bone Density that happens during aging can be slowed with *regular* physical activity.

These effects are seen in people who participate in aerobic, muscle-strengthening, and bone-strengthening physical activity programs of moderate or vigorous intensity.

The range of *total physical activity* for these benefits varies widely. Important changes seem to begin at *90 minutes a week* and continue up to *300 minutes a week*.

Lower Cancer Risk

Physically active people have a significantly lower risk of Colon cancer than do inactive people, and physically active women have a significantly lower risk of Breast cancer. The main reason for these benefits is that constant and consistent Physical Activity 'Burns" off the Energy from food and Uses and Expends it BEFORE it has a chance to collect and form into Adipose Tissue.

Research shows that a range of *moderate-intensity* physical activity—between *210 and 420 minutes a week* (3 hours and 30 minutes to 7 hours)—is needed to *significantly reduce* the risk of colon and breast cancer; currently, *150 minutes a week does not provide a major benefit*.

It also appears that greater amounts of physical activity lower risks of these cancers even further, although exactly how much lower is not clear.

Although not definitive, some research suggests that the risk of Endometrial cancer in women and Lung cancers in men and women also may be *lower* among those who are regularly active compared to those who are inactive.

Finally, cancer survivors have a *better quality of life* and *improved physical fitness* if they are physically *active*, compared to survivors who are inactive.

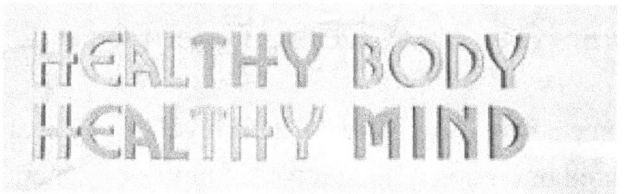

Mental Health

Physically active adults have *lower risk* of depression and cognitive decline (declines with aging in thinking, learning, and judgment skills). ***Motion generates more Electro-Magnetic Energy that is needed to produce, maintain and express the Highest Qualities of Humanity!***

Mental health benefits have been found in people who do Aerobic or a combination of Aerobic and muscle-strengthening activities 3 to 5 days a week for 30 to 60 minutes at a time. Some research has shown that even lower levels of physical activity also may provide some benefits.

Regular physical activity appears to reduce symptoms of anxiety and depression for children and adolescents as well as improve the quality of sleep, distress and anxiety in adults.

There is significant research that supports that physical activity significantly improves self-esteem.

The Brain requires approximately 20% of every Breath we Inhale. Aerobic or Cardiovascular exercises increases the amount of Oxygen intake which allows the Brain to be fully Charged and allow for the Manifesting of High Thoughts and decreases the potential for low quality thoughts like Depression, distress, anxiety and Low self-esteem.

Lower Risk of Adverse Events

Some people hesitate to become active or to increase their level of physical activity because they fear getting injured or having a heart attack. Studies of generally healthy people clearly show that moderate-intensity physical activity, such as brisk walking, has a low risk of such adverse events.

The risk of Musculoskeletal injury increases with the total amount of physical activity. For example, a person who regularly runs 40 miles a week has a higher risk of injury than a person who runs 10 miles each week.

However, people who are physically active may have fewer injuries from other causes, such as motor vehicle collisions or work-related injuries. Depending on the type and amount of activity that physically active people do, their overall injury rate may be lower than the overall injury rate for inactive people.

Participation in contact or collision sports, such as soccer or football, has a higher risk of injury than participation in noncontact physical activity, such as swimming or walking. However, when performing the same activity, people who are less fit are more likely to be injured than people who are more fit.

Cardiac events, such as a heart attack or sudden death during physical activity, are rare. However, the risk of such cardiac events does increase when a person suddenly becomes much more active than usual.

The greatest risk occurs when an adult who is usually inactive engages in vigorous-intensity activity (such as shoveling snow).

People who are regularly physically active have the lowest risk of cardiac events both while being active and overall.

The bottom line is that the health benefits of physical activity far outweigh the risks of adverse events for almost everyone.

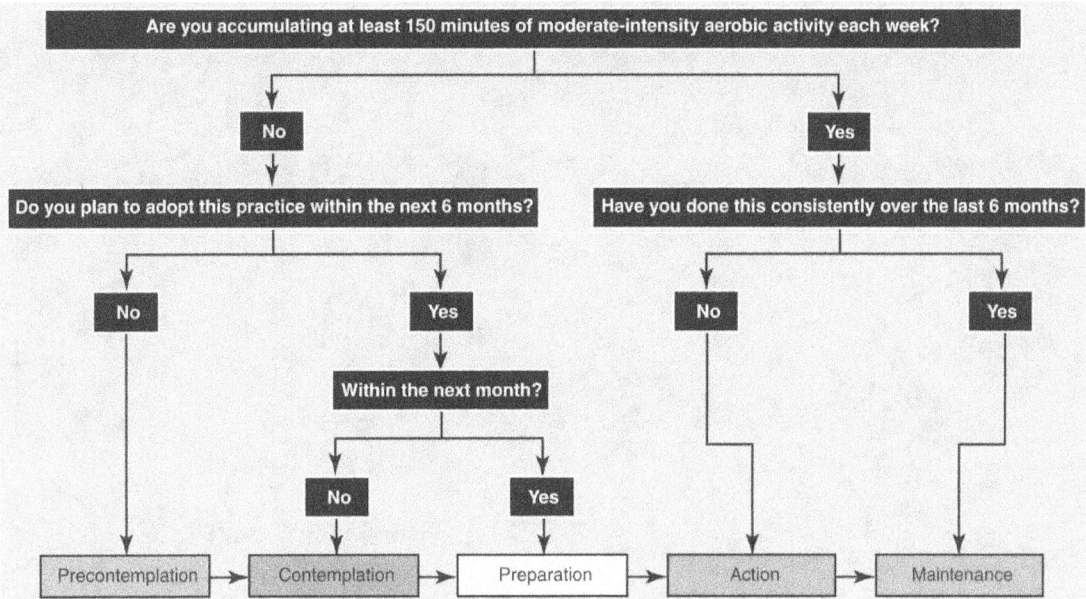

People who spent at least 6 hours of their daily leisure time sitting died sooner than people who sat less than 3 hours, according to a 14-year study.

Those who sit a lot and exercise little are at even greater risk of death.

Researchers found that sitting for that length of time by itself was detrimental to health. Sitting increased the risk of cancer death, but the main death risk linked to sitting was heart disease.

Sedentary individuals should be encouraged to stand up and walk around. Reaching optimal levels of physical exercise should also be encouraged.

The "Four Horsemen" of bad health—*poor diet*, *inactivity*, *smoking*, and *excessive drinking*—may indeed add up to a personal apocalypse, researchers have found.

Mortality risk rose 85% for individuals with any one of these risky health behaviors and jumped nearly 3.5 times for those who engaged in all four vices, according to University of Oslo researchers.

Piling up all four unhealthy behaviors prematurely aged a person 12 years in terms of death risk.

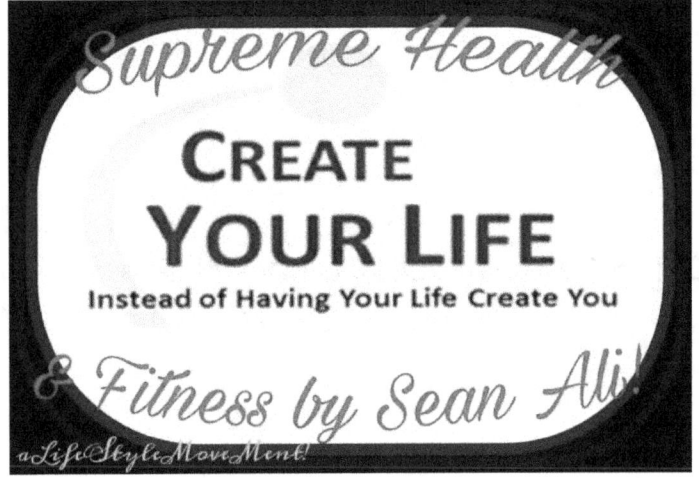

Critical Thinking

1.   If I help YOU to Eliminate YOUR Causes of Death ... What are YOU left with??

2.   How Long Do You Want To Live??

Chapter 7 ...

Changing to a Healthy LifeStyle!

*****

In adopting healthy behaviors (e.g., regular physical activity) or eliminating unhealthy ones (e.g., eating saturated fat), people progress through five stages related to their readiness for change.

At each stage, different intervention strategies help them progress to the next stage.

The Five distinct stages are:

1.   Precontemplation

2.   Contemplation

3.   Preparation

4.   Action

5.   Maintenance

Progression through the stages of change is *cyclical* rather than *linear*. Rarely does a person successfully go through the stages sequentially without encountering setbacks.

 Most people will recycle through the stages several times before being successful.

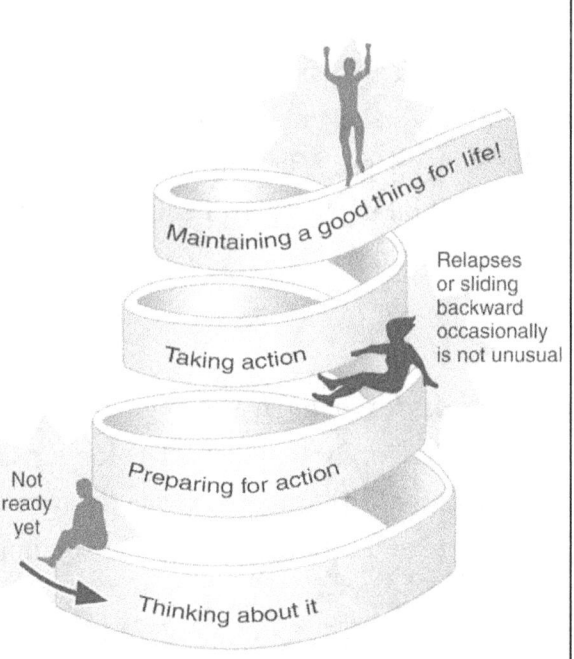

Stages of Change

1. *Precontemplation*: In this stage, the individual is recognizing a need to change and begins developing the thought about changing an unhealthy behavior in the next 6 months but is often caught between wanting to change and denying the need to change.

2. *Contemplation*: The individual is seriously thinking about changing an unhealthy behavior within the next 6 months. The thought-pattern becomes more focused on the need to change and the Will Power is significantly increasing to Move the Body to make manifest the Thought of Change into a Reality of Actual Change.

3. *Preparation*: This is considered a transitional stage in which the individual intends to take action within the next month. Some plans have been made, and the individual tries to determine what to do next.

4. *Action*: This stage is viewed as the 6 months following the overt modification and change of an unhealthy behavior. Motivation and investment in behavior change are sufficient in this stage, but it is the busiest and least stable stage and has the highest risk of relapse. The relapse is usually Mentally based, with the exception being from the result of an injury. Thinking there isn't enough time is the main excuse, followed closely by 'I don't know what to do.'

5. *Maintenance*: Maintenance begins after the individual has successfully adhered to the healthy behavior for 6 months. The longer someone stays in maintenance, the lower the risk of relapse. The longer the Maintenance stage the more the activities become 'second-nature' and a part of our Muscle Memory and daily routine.

Stage 1: Precontemplation

Precontemplation is the stage in which you are considering making a change in your life in the foreseeable future. Others in this stage have tried to change the past, failed, and simply given up.

Many of us know that it is important to make healthy choices, but in a world full of temptations and unhealthy alternatives it is often difficult to find the strength to make those changes in our lives.

Common excuses/obstacles to Living a Healthy Lifestyle

People often find it difficult to adhere to a healthy lifestyle of self-control because of:

■ Firmly established habits

■ Immediate gratification—people often want instant results or pleasure

■ Delayed negative health consequences of an unhealthy lifestyle—it may take years or even decades before the effects are seen

■ Invincibility—"it won't happen to me" belief in which it is assumed that poor health happens to others but not me; prefer dealing with life by taking risks or playing the odds that they will not contract a disease or get injured

■ Too much scientific information, which sometimes overwhelms or confuses

■ Fear of failure—often based on past failed attempts

■ Feeling a loss of control over one's life

■ Too many choices from which to pick for type of exercise, food, and weight control

Processes of Change	Stages of Change	Examples of Techniques
Consciousness-raising: increased awareness	Precontemplation Contemplation	Read news stories or a book; watch a TV program; talk with a friend or doctor
Social liberation: societal support for the healthy behavior change	Precontemplation Contemplation Preparation Action	Availability of a health club; restaurants offering low-fat/low-carb foods
Helping relationships: support system of family, friends, and co-workers	All five stages	Discuss your plans with others; join with another who is working on the behavior
Emotional arousal: emotional experience related to the unhealthy behavior	Contemplation Preparation	Personal testimony of someone who has solved a similar behavioral problem; seeing someone suffering the harmful consequences of his or her unhealthy behavior
Self-reevaluation: understanding that your behavior is how you are known	Contemplation Preparation	See yourself as fit
Commitment: making a firm commitment to change and believing that it can be done	Preparation Action Maintenance	Make a New Year's resolution; tell others about your intentions
Reward: increasing the rewards for positive behavioral change and decreasing the rewards for unhealthy behavior	Action Maintenance	Reward the behavior change (e.g., buying new clothes, movie ticket)
Countering: substituting healthy behavior for an unhealthy behavior	Action Maintenance	Take a walk instead of watching TV
Environmental control: avoiding triggers or using cues	Action Maintenance	Avoid dessert parties; leave encouraging messages on a calendar or stuck to the mirror or refrigerator

Precontemplation	Contemplation	Preparation	Action	Maintenance
Consciousness-Raising ——→				
Social Liberation ——————————————→				
Helping Relationships ————————————————————————→				
	Emotional Arousal ——→			
	Self-Reevaluation ——→			
		Commitment ————————————————→		
			Reward ——→	
			Countering ————→	
			Environmental Control ——→	

Stage 2: Contemplation

The Contemplation Stage occurs when you are aware that a problem exists and are seriously thinking about overcoming it, but have not yet made a commitment to take action. This is a time of reflection. Finding the reasons to change, the motivation to reach a goal, and the strength to make a plan work requires a lot of soul-searching.

This stage can take a good amount of time and should not be rushed. As important as it is to make a healthy change in your life, take the time to find what truly motivates you and your behavior.

This stage is the key to a successful course of action.

What Helps Change a Lifestyle?

Factors that influence an individual to change may include:

■ *Increasing knowledge*—this can influence one's behavior, but often may not be enough to influence people to change. The maxim "Why do we do what we do, when we know what we know?" illustrates that knowledge often is insufficient to affect behavior.

■   ***Motivation- having a reason***—a person may want to change to avoid sickness, to look and feel better, to live longer, or because of pressure from a spouse, child, or friend.

■   ***Readiness***—motivation is required, but may involve physical capabilities as well. Another maxim—"You can lead a horse to water, but you can't make it drink"—may reflect a lack of motivation or perhaps the physical inability to act for a variety reasons.

■   ***Landmark events***—resolutions to change often occur at the start of a new year, during a personal health crisis, on a birthday, upon the birth of a child, or the death of someone close to you.

■   ***Self-management techniques***—the ability to employ them helps individuals to make lifestyle changes.

Motivation

Motivation is what drives us to make changes. No matter how big or how small the change may be, we must be inspired to make choices. Finding what inspires or motivates you is an essential step in making a successful adjustment in your lifestyle.

The Level of Motivation directly determines the Level of Change!

Motivations for change could include:

■   Improving self-image and/or self-esteem

■   Being a role model for someone else

■   Improving relationships with family and peers

■   Reducing stress

■   Reducing risk of disease

Locus of Control

Life sometimes can involve many struggles for Control. Sometimes these struggles can manifest from external factors that can control or fight to control aspects of your life for a moment.

At other times the Power is seemingly IN your own hands. A significant key factor to successful change is locating what controls a certain behavior.

A **Locus of Control** is the figurative place where a person locates the source of responsibility in his or her life. This can manifest either externally or internally.

An External Locus of Control could be:

■ Believing others' actions determine your actions

■ Environmental factors—weather, location, and so on

■ Another person or social group

■ Blaming outside influences for your behavior

An Internal Locus of Control might be:

■ Self-expectations

■ Internal thoughts ("I can do this")

■ How open one is to change

To create a Successful Change in your life, YOU must be the one who takes the Responsibility for YOUR actions while simultaneously developing methods for overcoming any and all external barriers.

Individuals with an internal Locus of Control are more likely to see their behavior as something they can adapt or change.

If you not only Believe – but KNOW that it is within YOUR abilities alone, you may experience Greater Success!

Stage 3: Preparation

The Preparation phase combines Intention and Behavior to equal SUCCESS!

Here you will *monitor* your current behavior, *analyze* and *identify* patterns in your activity, and then *set* a goal. The most important concept in this stage is *Honesty*.

It is easy to try to make your behavior fit a certain pattern or profile. Sometimes the truth isn't what we want to see, but it is *imperative* to set realistic goals in order to achieve realistic changes.

When in the Preparation Stage, most individuals are intending to take action immediately within the next 30 days.

Self-Monitoring

Self-monitoring means *observing* and *recording* one's own behavior.

This process is necessary to:

■ Make you *aware* of the *size* and *seriousness* of a problem

■ Provide a benchmark to compare your original behavior (the point at which you began to try to change) with your later behavior

Behaviors need recording as they occur, not days later.

Self-monitoring devices to measure the frequency of a behavior include:

■ A health notebook, journal, or diary to record the occurrence of a behavior

■ Counters to collect data (e.g., pedometers, golf counters)

■ Graph paper (horizontal axis represents time—usually days—and vertical axis represents the amount of the behavior to be changed—body weight, exercise, number of hours of sleep)

Analysis

Once you have gathered your data, sit back and review your record. You are looking for patterns or clues about why and how you engage in the unhealthy behavior you wish to change. ***You should look at the following***:

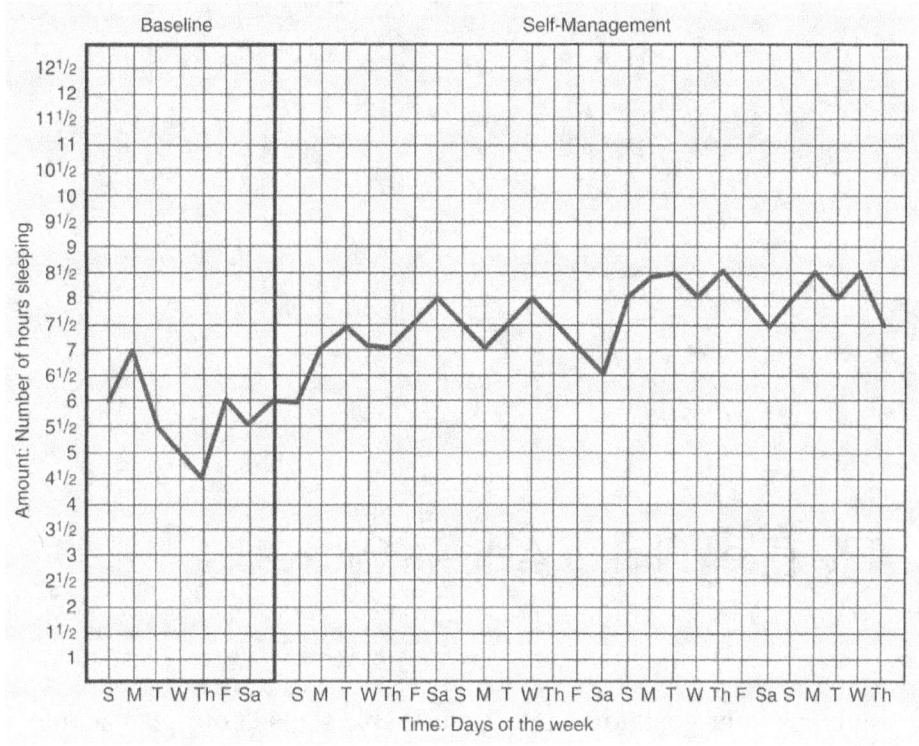

■   **Time.** When during the day or week do you find yourself resorting to the activity? Is it linked with another activity (e.g., smoking after a meal or with a beer)?

■   **Place.** Is there a specific place that you tend to be during the activity (e.g., making unhealthy diet choices on the way to class)?

■   **Reason.** Can you link the behavior with a mood or an event that might trigger it (e.g., indulging in comfort food before an exam)?

Sometimes these aspects may not be immediately clear. Take a few days to look over your log.

Remember that you are analyzing your behavior, not you as an individual.

Keep a positive outlook—this behavior may be less than perfect, but you are making strides to change it, and that is more than the majority can say!

The Easy Plan to Achieve Success!

The plan is where you break your goal down into manageable steps. Your plan should include:

■	What you will need. Do you need a newly stocked cabinet with healthier food? Do you need a gym membership? What equipment will you need for each of your steps?

■	What is your timeline? When will you start this plan? When is your ending date for your goal?

■	The steps you will take. Your goal should be broken down into smaller mini goals, each with its own timeline.

Easy Goal Setting to Achieve Success!

At this point, you have determined the where, when, and why for your behavior in question. The next step is to set a goal. Don't rush through this step. Certain factors must be taken into consideration for this goal to be effective

■ **Realistic.** While it is good to aim high, watch out for making your goal a bit too ambitious. If you set an unrealistic goal, you will become frustrated along the way and lose your motivation quickly. Aim for a moderate expectation—one that will challenge you but is within your ability. Remember that you can always set a higher goal once you reach this one.

■ **Quantitative.** Many times people set goals that are very abstract (i.e., wanting to lose weight). That is a fine ambition, but it is not an effective goal. You want your goal to be quantitative so that you can track your progress. A more effective goal would be to lose 10 pounds, or to stretch for 30 minutes three times a week. Try to define your goal in some type of measurable unit: minutes, pounds, number of servings, percentages, quantities, and so on.

■ **Broken down in steps.** If you start out thinking that you are aiming toward this one big goal from the beginning, you will find that it is easy to get discouraged during the first few weeks. You need to choose a goal that can be broken down into smaller intermediate steps—mini goals—along the way. For example, if the goal is to stop drinking soda, perhaps the mini goals could be to cut back to three sodas per day, then two, then one, and so on. Make sure your mini goals are quantitative.

■ **Tracked on a timeline.** Having the ambition to live a healthy lifestyle is different than trying to achieve your goal. The ambition can be carried with you for as long as you want. The goal, however, must have an end date. By using a timeline it is easier to keep your progress on track. The end date is not the end of the healthy behavior. After you have completed your goal within the time frame you chose, be sure to continue practicing the healthy habits until they stick!

■ **Important to you.** If you do not feel that this goal is important or worthwhile, it will not be a success. It does not matter how many people tell you that your goal is great, you have to believe in it yourself. If you don't, go back and revise the goal until it fits with your expectations and your motivation.

The Easy Contract to Achieve Success!

Write a contract binding Yourself to the chosen course of action. It should be one that You can easily adhere to and that guarantees Your Success!

Your contract should include:

- **Start date:** Write the date that you will begin your plan.

- **Finish date:** Write the date when you will have completed your goal.

- **The Goal:** Be specific and concise.

- **Motivation (benefits):** Determine what is in it for you.

- **Identify your current stage of change.**

- **Identify the processes (strategies) of change:** Use <u>Figure 3.3</u> for each possible stage of change.

- **For each process of change to be used, identify a specific technique.**

- **Identify the stage of change when you finish.**

- **Mini goals with rewards:** What are the intervals along the way that will indicate you are making progress?

- **Your signature:** Sign your name as a sign of your commitment to your plan.

- **Witness signature:** Have a close friend or family member sign your contract as well.

PERSONAL CONTRACT

Start Date: _____ Finish Date: _____

The Goal: _____

Motivation (benefits): _____

Identify your current stage of change: _____

Match your current stage of change and other stages you anticipate progressing through with the appropriate processes of change (see Figure 3.3):

_____   _____

_____   _____

What specific techniques will you use for each of the processes identified above (see Table 1.1)?	
Processes	Specific techniques
Stage of change on the finish date:	

Mini goals	Date	Reward
_____	_____	_____
_____	_____	_____
_____	_____	_____

I, _____, agree to work toward a healthier lifestyle and in doing so shall comply with the terms and dates of this contract.

Signature: _____ Date: _____

Witness: _____ Date: _____

Stage 4: Action

The Action Stage is where you begin to Consciously Move toward a Healthier Behavior. You have *Your Motivation, Your Internal Locus Of Control*, and *Your Goal*.

You are ready to make this change!

Action involves the most observable behavioral changes and requires the greatest commitments of Time and Energy.

It is important to be mindful that sometimes your Energy level during the action phase can dwindle down, leaving the success of your plan vulnerable to barriers.

The five main barriers to successful change are:

- Social impact

- Stress

- Postponing

- Justification

- Denying responsibility

Social Impact

During this Stage, there can be both Positive and Negative social impacts on Your Plan to change a behavior. Knowing or able to identify bot can help you Strengthen your Resolve, effectively avoid pit-falls while simultaneously recognizing potential benefits.

Positive social impacts may be in the form of:

- Structured support groups

- Cheerleading by friends and family

- Role models—people around you whom you respect and admire

Negative social impacts may include:

■   Feeling like the odd one out

■   Peer pressure

■   Attending functions that tempt you to break your contract

A good catalyst for Success is to let those around you know that you are trying to change this specific behavior. They may be able to offer tips and suggestions to help you along. More importantly, if you explain your goals to them, they are more likely to respect your decision and less likely to pressure you into relapsing into old behavior patterns.

Stress

One of the biggest barriers to changing lifestyle behaviors is **Stress**. Stress can occur anywhere in our daily lives and without the correct management techniques it can lead you away from your goal.

Cellular Adaptation to Injury or Stress

Injury or Stress	Adaptation
Increased demand ⟶	Hyperplasia or hypertrophy
Decreased stimulation or lack of nutrients ⟶	Atrophy
Chronic irritation ⟶	Metaplasia

Eating comfort food, drinking, and engaging in other reckless behavior are common ways that many people deal with stress—none of which are effective or healthy.

Learning effective coping techniques can make it easier for you to stay on track with your plan of action and help you to create a better sense of wellness overall.

Postponement

After that initial surge of motivation in the beginning of the action phase, it can get difficult to muster the necessary Energy to continue to make the healthy choices. Many times the steps to reaching your goal get pushed aside or postponed until a later point in time. It is best to stop the **Procrastination** as soon as you feel yourself slipping into that mindset.

When you realize that you are postponing a step in your plan:

■   Stop and identify ***out loud*** that you are Procrastinating. It makes a lot of difference and easily accepted when hearing Your Own voice recognizing Your Own Truth bout Your Own Choices versus the same information coming from someone else. We Can't Lis To OURSELVES!

■   Try to pin down why you are avoiding that particular step. For example, is cold weather causing you to avoid going to the gym? Or is that healthy dish too time-consuming to make?

■   Once you have identified why you are postponing a particular step, try to revise that step to fit better with your life. For example, buy a few exercise DVDs for working out at home when the weather is bad. Or, find simpler recipes that still offer the same nutritional value.

Justification

Many times when we procrastinate we justify or **Rationalize** our actions. We make excuses for why we have not completed the task.

It is important to catch yourself if you find that you are justifying not meeting your goal or one of your steps.

Your plan may quickly become a slippery slope where nothing is accomplished, but everything is rationalized.

When you feel yourself making excuses:

■   Say your excuse out loud and listen—is it credible?

■   Write down those times when you push your task off and explain why you did so. If you find yourself falling off course with your goal, these logs will provide a good resource describing when and why you aren't meeting each step.

■   Understand that there will be times when you can't complete a step that second. Make sure that you are justifying the valid procrastinations, not the ones made out of low motivation.

Denying Responsibility

Along with justification can come **Blaming**. Blaming occurs when You displace the responsibility for missing a step or not completing a goal onto someone else (external locus of control).

Because of *him/her/them* or what *they* did, the goal was not met.

This is an easy trap to fall into because it is convenient and gives the appearance that YOU are not at fault.

BUT No matter how good blaming looks on paper, it will not help you reach your goal.

 You will still be left with an unfinished plan.

It is important to accept responsibility for your own actions.

Stage 5: Maintenance

After at least 6 months in the Action Stage, the person may successfully transition into the fifth stage: Maintenance.

This phase is when you keep up the new healthier habits that have replaced the old habits without much worry of returning to the old behavior.

Change is maintained more easily now. There may be an initial excitement associated with making a change in which your motivation and commitment will both be high and the outlook toward your goal is positive.

Many of the activities used in the maintenance phase are the same as you'll use if you are in the action phase, just with small adaptations. For instance:

■   **Rewards:** You still need to set reward dates; however, they are more distant and the rewards should become smaller as the behavior becomes more natural.

■   **Environmental control:** Once the first set of influences is overcome, new challenges can be established.

Common Issues to Face in Maintenance

Relapse

Relapse can occur at any *stage* of the Change process. It can be triggered by many things: an extra stressful day or week, an unexpected event, low levels of motivation. If you find yourself *relapsing* along the way, try to *identify* a reason. Are you losing motivation?

Is your plan unrealistic?

Do you not have the right equipment or facilities?

This is a *Process*, which means that nothing is set in stone. You have the freedom to go back and revise your goal at any time. ***Don't be afraid to reevaluate your plan***.

If something is not working for you, find alternatives that will still help you successfully change the unwanted negative behavior.

Most importantly: Do not give up!

A relapse is normal—it doesn't mean that you will never complete your goals. It is a minor setback that can be overcome.

Acceptance

Acceptance is the finish line.

The old unhealthy behavior has been fully replaced at this point. Not only have you completed your Goal, but you have also integrated other important and necessary Healthy habits into your daily routine.

Be aware that this stage may not come quickly.

Achieving your goal and dealing with relapses may take a long while, but your healthy new lifestyle is definitely worth it and You Will Be Able To Successfully Enjoy Abundant Life!

- All adults should avoid inactivity. Some physical activity is better than none, and adults who participate in any amount of physical activity gain some health benefits.

- For substantial health benefits, adults should do at least 150 minutes (2 hours and 30 minutes) a week of moderate-intensity, or 75 minutes (1 hour and 15 minutes) a week of vigorous-intensity aerobic physical activity, or an equivalent combination of moderate- and vigorous-intensity aerobic activity. Aerobic activity should be performed in episodes of at least 10 minutes, and preferably, it should be spread throughout the week.

- For additional and more extensive health benefits, adults should increase their aerobic physical activity to 300 minutes (5 hours) a week of moderate-intensity, or 150 minutes a week of vigorous-intensity aerobic physical activity, or an equivalent combination of moderate- and vigorous-intensity activity. Additional health benefits are gained by engaging in physical activity beyond this amount.

- Adults should also do muscle-strengthening activities that are moderate or high intensity and involve all major muscle groups on 2 or more days a week, as these activities provide additional health benefits.

Critical Thinking

1. If I help YOU to Eliminate YOUR Causes of Death ... What are YOU left with??

2. How Long Do You Want To Live??

Chapter 8 ....

Successfully Over-Coming Stress!

*****

What Is Stress?

Stress can be broadly defined as an automatic physical response to any stimulus that requires you to adjust to change.

Good stress is referred to as **Eustress** and helps you perform better and overcome obstacles.

Bad stress is referred to as **Distress** and upsets you and makes you sick.

Chronic or overabundant stress wears down the ability to adapt and cope – expressed in the figure below.

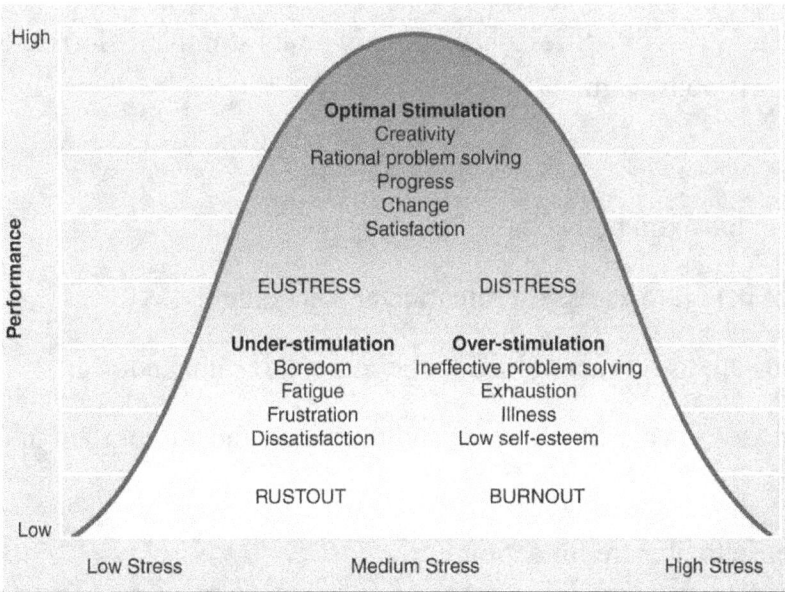

The Stress Continuum showing the effects of stress on performance.

You feel distressed if you believe that:

- You have more problems than you can handle.

- You don't feel up to a task.

Identifying Your Stressors

Exercising until you are exhausted is a *Physical Stressor*.

Taking a tough exam is a *Mental Stressor*.

Giving an in-class report is a *Social Stressor*.

Being in a room filled with loud music is an *Environmental Stressor.*

How you respond to the stressor is known as your *Stress Response*.

How Does Your Body Respond to Stress?

In the natural response to Stress or a Stressor, your body pours stimulant Hormones, such as Adrenaline, into your Bloodstream.

The effects are:

- You sweat to cool the extra body heat.

- You hear and see better, to assess the situation and act quickly.

- Your heart speeds up, to get more blood to the muscles, brain, and heart.

- Blood flow increases to your brain, heart, and muscles—most important in dealing with danger.

- Your muscles tense to prepare for action.

- Less blood flows to your skin, digestive tract, kidneys and liver—least needed in times of crisis.

- You breathe faster, to take in more oxygen.

- Your liver dumps extra sugar and fats into your bloodstream for quick energy.

- Platelets and blood-clotting factors rise to prevent hemorrhage in case of injury.

How Does Your Nervous System React to Stress?

The **Sympathetic Nervous Subsystem** of the **Autonomic Nervous System** triggers the necessary Energy output to handle a specific or perceived crisis, including Stress. These responses acts on many parts of the body, such as Sweat Glands, Blood Vessels, and Muscles.

Endorphins: Pain-inhibiting Brain secretions.

Sympathetic Nervous System: Subsystem of the Autonomic system that triggers your body's response to Stress—known as the *Fight-or-Flight* response.

Autonomic Nervous System: Part of the Nervous System that controls *automatic* body functions, such as *blood pressure*, *heart rate*, and *breathing*. This system is subdivided into the *Sympathetic* and *Parasympathetic* systems.

How Does Your Endocrine System React to Stress?

Your **Endocrine System** releases **Hormones** to *control* body functions. It's the system that your body uses to communicate with itself.

In response to a Stressor, it releases extra Hormones from the Adrenal **Glands** and Pituitary Gland, giving rise to the Stress response.

What Is the Fight-or-Flight Response?

The **Stress Hormones** (Epinephrine, Norepinephrine, Cortisol) secreted into the Bloodstream prepare the body for *quick action* during times of Stress.

This particular Stress Response is often called "*Fight-or-Flight*" because it gets you ready to take action either by staying and fighting or by running away from danger. Even in situations not necessarily requiring a physical response (e.g., being late for an in-class exam, having to stop at three red lights in a row, being unable to find a parking space), the *Fight-or-Flight* response may still be activated, releasing the same Chemical Hormone re-action.

How Do You Return to Normal?

Once you have stopped the Stressing process over something, the Parasympathetic Subsystem of your Autonomic Nervous System takes over and starts the reversal process of Calming you down. This process takes you back to **Homeostasis** by bringing down your Blood Pressure, Heart Rate, and Hormone levels; drying your sweaty palms; and slowing your breathing back to a normal pace.

Common Personality Types Associated to Stress

There are certain kinds of behavior that can aggravate the effects of Stress. These behaviors are commonly grouped into 2 categories – *Type A* and *Type B*

Extreme **type-A** people are at *risk* of coronary problems, unless they become able to channel their drive in *constructive* ways and keep themselves in good physical shape.

Type-B: people take things easy, do not respond to pressure or hurry, and do not set deadlines for themselves. They have a *secure* sense of Self-Esteem.

However, an *extreme* type-B person may be *avoiding* life's challenges and as a result may *not* accomplish much.

Endocrine system: Consists of Glands that produce Hormones that *control* body functions.

Hormone: Chemical messenger released into the Bloodstream that *controls* many body activities.

Gland: A group of Cells that secretes Hormones.

Stress Hormones (e.g., epinephrine): A Hormone that prepares the body to react during times of stress or in an emergency.

Homeostasis: Stability and consistency of a person's Physiology.

Type A: An individual exhibiting a sense of time urgency ("hurry sickness"), aggressiveness, and competitiveness, usually combined with hostility. *Describes a great majority of Americans.*

Type B: An individual displaying no sense of time urgency, no hostility, non-competitiveness, patience, and a secure sense of self-esteem.

Common Unhealthy Responses to Stress

Behavioral Responses

- Pacing and fidgeting, nail-biting, foot-tapping

- Overeating or weight gain, insufficient food, or underweight

- Smoking, drinking too much, taking illegal or unsafe drugs

- Taking prescription or over-the-counter drugs that promise some form of relief such as muscle relaxants, sleeping pills, or anti-anxiety pills

- Crying, yelling, swearing, blaming other people and things

- Throwing things or hitting someone

- Watching endless hours of TV

- Sleeping too much

Mental Responses

- Decreased concentration and memory

- Mind racing or going blank, confusion, indecisiveness

- Loss of sense of humor

Emotional Responses

- Anger and frustration, short temper, irritability, impatience

- Anxiety, nervousness, worry, fear

- Boredom, general fatigue, depression, low self-esteem

Stress and Dis-ease

Of all illnesses, 50% to 80% relate to stress. **The top-selling drugs in the United States are for stress-related disorders**.

According to the American Academy of Family Physicians, two-thirds of all medical office visits are for stress-related illnesses.

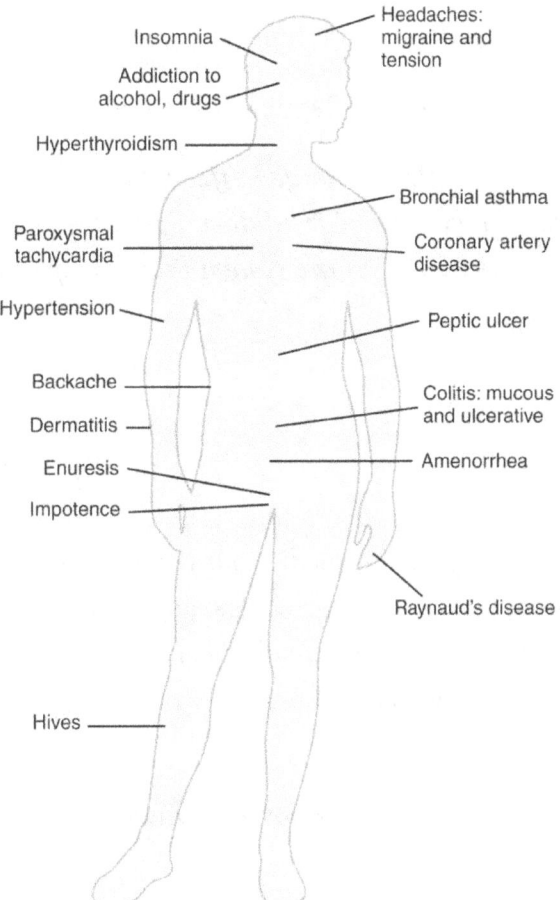

Insomnia

Addiction to alcohol, drugs

Hyperthyroidism

Headaches: migraine and tension

Bronchial asthma

Paroxysmal tachycardia

Coronary artery disease

Hypertension

Peptic ulcer

Backache

Colitis: mucous and ulcerative

Dermatitis

Enuresis

Amenorrhea

Impotence

Raynaud's disease

Hives

Psychoneuroimmunology

Depending on your body's and mind's ability to cope with stress, you can develop some serious health problems as a result of *Chronic Stress*, especially in your Circulatory and Immune systems:

- High blood pressure and arteriosclerosis leading to stroke or heart attack

- Increased susceptibility to colds, infections, rheumatoid arthritis, cancer, herpes, HIV

Other health problems from poor response to stress can include:

- Rapid or irregular heart rate, chest pains

- Muscle aches or stiffness (especially in neck, shoulders, and low back)

- Temporomandibular joint dysfunction

- Tension or migraine headaches

- Flushing or sweating, trembling, fatigue, cold extremities

- Nausea, abdominal cramps, irritable bowel syndrome, ulcers, and colitis

- Bronchial asthma, allergies, insomnia

Stress is deadly in the prolonged effects that cause almost irreparable damage to our 2 Major Life systems – the Circulatory System that is responsible for the distribution of Life Energy and the Immune system that is responsible for Self-Healing, Repair and Regeneration.

Healthy Diet

What you eat plays a big role in your risk of developing many illnesses, including hypertension, heart disease, diabetes, and cancer, which in turn affect your overall stress level. Obesity caused by overeating is linked with many ailments, too. It is also a source of stress for those who are continually reminded of their failure to achieve the slim look desired in America.

The act of eating has only 2 possible outcomes = we are Eating to Die or EATING TO LIVE!

- Eat a well-balanced diet of milk, whole grains, fruits, vegetables; eat slowly; NO junk food, juices or sodas.

- Take in less caffeine (e.g., coffee, tea, colas, too much chocolate). Caffeine *generates* a Stress Reaction in the body.

- Avoid "stress-reducing" supplements, such as those containing vitamins and amino acid compounds. *They do not help reduce the effects of stress.*

Exercise

Exercise is a good way to dissipate stress. Get regular exercise (at least 30 minutes, three times per week). Take a brisk walk, a run, or a bike ride.

Cardiovascular exercise flushes stress hormones out of the body. Otherwise, they pool in the body and cause havoc (e.g., cortisol destroys white blood cells). Regular cardiovascular exercise may contribute to an overall sense of relaxation.

Exercise may also combat emotional problems, such as depression, by increasing the level of endorphins, chemicals in the brain that seem to enhance a sense of well-being and relieve anxiety.

Sleep

Sleep **reduces** Stress. Tired people do not cope well with stressful situations. If you get enough sleep, you feel better and are more resilient and adaptable.

The act of sleep or Resting is when a majority of the regenerative process is performed. We have less things that our attention/Energy is focused on, so the Body can focus/concentrate on Healing Self!

Successful sleep is:

- Waking naturally

- Waking refreshed

- Having plenty of daytime energy

The "power nap" or catnap is short (5 to 20 minutes) and can be rejuvenating. Many people don't get enough sleep, some by choice. But bad things happen when you are sleep deprived:

- You doze off in class.

- You can't focus on an exam.

- You risk serious injury by dozing off while driving or working.

Lack of sleep also adversely affects your health:

■   You are at a greater risk of infection.

■   You become moody.

■   You have problems with memory.

When do you Know that you are getting enough sleep?

When you wake up naturally without an alarm clock and feel alert during the day?

Defense Mechanism	Positive or Negative?	Definition	Simple Example
Affiliation	Positive	Sharing your feelings of stress, without trying to make others take responsibility for it.	Talking with a close friend about the difficulties you are having with speaking in front of class.
Humor	Positive	Finding the humor or irony of a situation. Differs from sarcasm, which is an anger response.	At the end of a day filled with conflict, finding humor in the ridiculous odds that "all those things" could happen in the same day.
Denial	Negative	Pretending a stressor is minor or does not exist.	Failing to recognize the possibility one has an alcohol problem after receiving a third DUI citation.
Rationalization	Negative	Defending or justifying personal actions and feelings others find unacceptable.	"I only smoke when I drink, so I'm not really a smoker."
Splitting	Negative	Categorization of others in one's life; idolizing one group and disenfranchising the other.	After a major argument with all four roommates, ignoring and shutting out those who disagreed with you, while spending all your time with those who did agree.
Repression	Negative	Blocking disturbing thoughts or experiences from the conscious mind.	Often used by those having experienced physical, emotional, or sexual abuse as children so the upsetting thoughts are not always present.

Additional Easy Ways to Manage Stress

Music

Listening to and creating music has a soothing effect. For most people, music is a popular way to relax. Individual tastes vary greatly regarding music. However, certain factors associated with music as a relaxation technique include the following:

■　　The music should be instrumental with a slow tempo. The music should be enjoyable rather than agitating.

■　　Minimize or eliminate all interruptions.

■　　Sit or recline in a comfortable position with eyes closed to minimize distractions.

■　　Make your own music by humming, singing, whistling a song, or playing an instrument.

Time-outs

Take time-outs to get away from the things that are bothering you. This will decrease your stress level.

Time-outs include power naps, meditation, daydreaming, a social conversation, a short walk, a refreshment break, or listening to music.

You have cycles throughout the day, peaks of energy and concentration interspersed with low energy and inefficiency. Watch for periods of low energy and take breaks when they occur.

A mid-morning break, lunch, a mid-afternoon break, and the evening meal divide a day into roughly 2-hour segments.

Get up 15 minutes earlier

Prepare for the morning the night before

Avoid tight-fitting clothes

Avoid relying on chemical aids

Set appointments ahead

Don't rely on your memory... write it down

Practice preventive maintenance

Make duplicate keys

Say "no" more often

Set priorities in your life

Avoid negative people

Use time wisely

Simplify mealtimes

Always make copies of important papers

Anticipate your needs

Repair anything that doesn't work properly

Ask for help with the jobs you dislike

Break large tasks into bite-size portions

Look at problems as challenges

Look at challenges differently

Unclutter your life

Smile

Be prepared for rain

Tickle a baby

Pet a friendly dog/cat

Don't know all the answers

Look for a silver lining

Say something nice to someone

Teach a kid to fly a kite

Walk in the rain

Schedule play time into every day

Take a bubble bath

Be aware of the decisions you make

Believe in yourself

Stop saying negative things to yourself

Visualize yourself winning

Develop your sense of humor

Stop thinking tomorrow will be a better today

Have goals for yourself

Dance a jig

Say "hello" to a stranger

Ask a friend for a hug

Look up at the stars

Practice breathing slowly

Learn to whistle a tune

Read a poem

Listen to a symphony

Watch a ballet

Read a story curled up in bed

Do a brand new thing

Stop a bad habit

Buy yourself a flower

Take time to smell the flowers

Find support from others

Ask someone to be your "vent-partner"

Do it today

Work at being cheerful and optimistic

Put safety first

Do everything in moderation

Pay attention to your appearance

Strive for excellence *not* perfection

Stretch your limits a little each day

Look at a work of art

Hum a jingle

Maintain your weight

Plant a tree

Feed the birds

Practice grace under pressure

Stand up and stretch

Always have a plan "B"

Learn a new doodle

Memorize a joke

Be responsible for your feelings

Learn to meet your own needs

Become a better listener

Know your limitations and let others know them, too

Tell someone to have a good day in pig Latin

Throw a paper airplane

Exercise every day

Learn the words to a new song

Get to work early

Clean out one closet

Play patty cake with a toddler

Go on a picnic

Take a different route to work

Leave work early (with permission)

Put air freshener in your car

Watch a movie and eat popcorn

Write a note to a faraway friend

Go to a ballgame and scream

Cook a meal and eat it by candlelight

Recognize the importance of unconditional love

Remember that stress is an attitude

Keep a journal

Practice a monster smile

Remember you always have options

Have a support network of people, places, and things

Quit trying to fix other people

Get enough sleep

Talk less and listen more

Freely praise other people

Bonus: Relax, take each day at a time ... you have the rest of your life to live!

Chapter 9 ...

Building Supreme Health!

*****

Physical Activity, Modern Civilization, and Chronic Disease

The Centers for Disease Control and Prevention (CDC) defines **Physical Activity** as any bodily movement produced by the Contraction of Skeletal Muscles that increases Energy Expenditure above a Basal level.

Examples of this type of physical activity would be walking or riding a bike as a form of transportation, using the stairs instead of the escalator, or manual labor such as carpentry work, gardening, or farming.

Physical Activity differs from **Exercise** based on it's **structure** and **purpose**.

Exercise is classified as a *subcategory* of Physical Activity that is sub-divided into 4 categories of *Planned*, *Structured*, *Repetitive*, and *Purposive* in the sense that the improvement or maintenance of one or more components of physical fitness is the objective. People engage in Exercise for the purpose of training, competing, and keeping organs and bodily functions healthy. Examples of exercise include aerobic classes, jogging, running, swimming, cycling, weight training, tennis, and other such bouts of planned activities with the intension of improving overall physical fitness.

Physical Fitness is defined by the CDC as the ability to carry out daily tasks with vigor and alertness, without undue fatigue, and with ample energy to enjoy leisure-time pursuits and respond to emergencies. Physical fitness includes a number of components consisting of cardiorespiratory endurance (aerobic power), skeletal muscle endurance, skeletal muscle strength, skeletal muscle power, flexibility, balance, speed of movement, reaction time, and body composition.

Physical inactivity is a global health problem and is estimated by the World Health Organization (WHO) to contribute to 3.2 million deaths annually. There are only three risk factors considered to contribute to mortality with a higher prevalence worldwide: **high blood pressure**, **tobacco use**, and **high blood glucose**.

Increased participation in regular physical activity as a part of everyday life remains a national health goal. The U.S. Department of Health and Human Services (USDHHS), in its report *Healthy People 2020* has set health-related goals for Americans in nutrition and physical fitness. The 2020 target is to reduce the percentage of adults who do not engage in any leisure-time physical activity to 32.6% or less. Current progress reports indicate that only 43.5% of adults meet the minimum recommendation of aerobic physical activity and muscle-strengthening activity on a regular basis. All *Healthy People 2020* objectives are available at www.healthypeople.gov/2020/.

A Body In Motion Stays In Motion

Nature of Energy

The term *Energy* refers to the Body's Ability, or Power, to Do Work. The Energy required to do work takes several different forms: Mechanical, Chemical, Electrical, Radiant, and Heat.

Energy, like matter, can **neither** be created nor destroyed. It can only be changed into another form; therefore, Energy is constantly cycled in the body and environment. We also speak of energy as being potential or kinetic.

Potential Energy is Stored Energy, ready to be used.

Kinetic Energy is Active Energy, being used to do work.

Energy Balance in physical activity requires appropriate nutrition to supply the substrate fuels, which along with oxygen and water, meet widely varying levels of energy demands for body action.

Regular endurance exercise can benefit the body in many healthy ways.

The following are the **Short**- and **Long**-term benefits achieved by exercising regularly, using the cardiorespiratory system.

Short-Term Benefits

Many people start a physical activity program because of its long-term benefits; however, it is the short-term benefits that keep them motivated to continue the habit.

Relaxes and Revitalizes

Physical activity **reduces** Mental and Muscular Tension and **increases** Concentration and Energy levels. Regular Aerobic exercise releases **<u>Endorphins</u>**.

Offers a Break from Daily Routine and Stress

Planned or unplanned physical activity can be enjoyable and provide a release from day-to-day stress and boredom.

Helps You Feel Good About Yourself

Physical activity can improve your self-esteem and self-confidence and enhance your general sense of well-being.

Long-Term Benefits

Decreases Risk of Heart Disease

The leading health threat today is cardiovascular disease, which includes heart attack, stroke, hypertension, coronary artery disease (the buildup of fatty deposits on the inside of arteries), and congestive heart failure. Coronary artery disease (also called heart disease) and stroke are major causes of disability.

Prevents plaque buildup in arteries.

Atherosclerosis is another key factor in Cardiovascular dis-ease. Fatty deposits called Plaques build-up as particles of low-density lipoprotein (LDL, or "bad" cholesterol) pass out of the bloodstream and lodge in weakened portions of artery walls, including the arteries supplying the heart and the brain.

Over time, these Plaques can **narrow** the Vessels enough to deprive these Organs of Oxygen-rich Blood. When this happens in the heart, it can lead to a Heart attack. Blocked Arteries in the Brain can result in a Stroke.

Moderate to vigorous aerobic exercise **increases** healthy High-Density Lipoprotein (HDL) Cholesterol in our blood. HDL transports Fats back to your Liver for Metabolism, preventing their **accumulation** along Artery walls. Exercise also significantly **reduces** the blood levels of **unhealthy** LDL Cholesterol and Triglycerides.

Protects Arteries.

Exercise can help keep arteries resilient. Regular expansion and contraction of arteries during exercise keeps the vessels "in shape." Arteries are the HIGHWAY for our Life Energy to travel throughout Self. Oxygen, the Breath Of Life is dispersed through our Arteries.

Makes clots less likely

Exercise helps keep the Inner-lining of the Arteries healthy and thereby less prone to injuries that set the stage for Plaque formation. It also **inhibits** Clot formation by making Platelets less "**sticky**" and **promotes** the release of the necessary Enzymes that break-down these Clots. Higher activity levels lower Inflammation in the Arteries.

Promotes new coronary arteries.

Aerobic exercise can lead to an **increase** in the Size and Number of Coronary Arteries **feeding** the Heart. If an Arterial blockage occurs, there is **less risk** of Heart Muscle damage because there are alternative channels to keep the Blood supply flowing.

Decreases Risk of Cancer

Exercise increases circulation and respiration, accelerates the movement of food through the bowels, improves energy metabolism and immune function, and affects hormone levels. All of these may help protect against most types of cancer.

Lowers Blood Pressure

Exercise helps protect you from Cardiovascular dis-ease in numerous ways. The less active you are, the more likely you are to develop Hypertension. Chronic Hypertension *doubles or triples* the risk for developing Congestive Heart failure and can lead to heart disease, brain hemorrhage, aortic aneurysms, kidney disease and failure, and damage to other organs.

Increases Stamina

Exercise may cause fatigue immediately after the activity. Over the long term, though, it will increase stamina and reduce fatigue.

Lowers Body Fat

Exercise can counter creeping weight gain. Approximately 70% of the Energy burned every day is taken up by normal Bodily Functions; the remaining 30% depends on our level of activity, so exercise choices certainly make a difference.

For people who are *already* overweight, Exercise is an *integral* part of any weight-loss program. The most effective way to *lose* weight is to *increase* your level of Activity and to *reduce* the Calories you consume.

Cutting back on Calories leads to faster weight loss than from exercising. *Because you need to burn 3500 calories to lose a single pound, it may take a few weeks of regular, moderate exercise to successfully do so. However, consuming 500 less calories a day will result in the loss of a pound a week.*

If you only cut back on calories, however, you are more likely to regain the weight lost.

That is because your body reacts to weight loss as if it were starving and, in response, slows its metabolism. When your metabolism slows, you burn less calories. Increasing your physical activity will counteract the Metabolic slow-down caused by reducing calories.

Exercise *raises* your Energy Expenditure while you are exercising and also while you are resting when the workout is done. *Pounds lost by increasing your activity level consist almost entirely of Fat.*

Improves Muscular Health

Aerobic exercise stimulates the **growth** of Blood Vessels and Capillaries in the muscles, providing for more **efficient** Oxygen delivery to the Muscles and helping to **remove** irritating Metabolic Waste products such as Lactic Acid. This can significantly **reduce** pain in those who have Fibromyalgia and chronic low-back pain.

Reduces the Number of Sick Days

Many studies report that people who exercise regularly are less susceptible to minor viral illnesses, such as colds or flu, because of an **improved** Immune system, which significantly improves and increases the natural abilities of Self-Healing, Repair and Regeneration

Decreases the Chance of Pre-mature Death

In 1986, results from the Harvard Alumni Health Study published in the *New England Journal of Medicine* for the first time, linked Exercise with **increased** Life-spans. Since then, additional research has supported this finding.

Decreases Cholesterol and Triglyceride Levels

High blood Cholesterol and Triglyceride levels increase the risk of Heart dis-ease. Regular exercise raises the level of good cholesterol (HDL), which may help to clear blood vessels and to lower the level of bad cholesterol (LDL).

Decreases the Risk of Diabetes

Untreated or poorly treated diabetes can lead to blindness, kidney disease, and the loss of limbs. It is also a major factor in heart disease and stroke.

All Cells need Sugar in the form of Glucose as a source of Energy. Insulin is a Hormone that's produced by the Pancreas and helps the Cells to extract Sugar from the Blood. When you have diabetes, your body is **unable** to make or **use** Insulin efficiently, so you have excess Sugar (glucose) in your Blood.

About 5% to 10% of people with Diabetes **cannot** make Insulin at all; this condition is called Type 1 Diabetes.

Type 2 Diabetes accounts for 90% to 95% of cases of Diabetes. In the Type 2 Diabetes cases, the Pancreas can pump out *more* Insulin for a time, but eventually it cannot keep up with the greater demand, and Blood Glucose levels *rise*.

Type 2 Diabetes CAN be successfully controlled by proper dietary choices and exercise, although medications or insulin may eventually be needed.

Exercise lowers modest amounts of Blood Glucose and boosts the body's sensitivity to insulin.

This can help control existing diabetes and, most important, stave off the onset of Type 2 Diabetes.

Decreases the Risk of Osteoporosis

Weight-bearing exercise is necessary to stimulate the growth of new bone tissue. When demands are put on a bone, it responds by becoming stronger and denser.

Any activity that works against gravity can potentially build bone. Examples of such activities include running, walking, weight lifting, and stair climbing. However, activities such as swimming or biking, which are not weight-bearing, do not build bone. Higher-impact activities or resistance exercises (e.g., strength training) have a greater effect on bone than lower-impact exercises (e.g., walking) do. Only the bone that actually bears the load of the exercise will benefit, however. For example, walking or running protects bones in the lower extremities. A well-rounded strength training plan can help all of your bones.

Decreases Arthritis Symptoms

Overuse of certain joints can set the stage for Arthritis, but *regular moderate activity* does *not* raise the risk for this dis-ease developing in normal Joints. *Instead*, moderate exercise—whether Aerobic or Resistance—actually *helps* to *reduce* swelling in Joints and *relieve* Pain.

When Joints are not used, the Cartilage *thins* and *softens*, making the Joint more *vulnerable* to Arthritis. Exercise can also *control* weight.

Overweight and **obesity** put people at a much higher risk for developing arthritis.

Muscle Physiology

Muscle Structure

There is a **synchronized action** of millions of **specialized** Cells that make up our Skeletal Muscle mass makes possible all forms of physical activity. A **finely coordinated** series of small bundles within the Muscle Fibers produce a smooth symphony of action through simultaneous and alternating **Contraction** and **Relaxation**.

These successively smaller muscle structures include the following:

• **Fasciculi**: A bundle of Muscle Fibers.

• **Muscle fiber**: Muscle Cells composed of bundles of still smaller Strands called *Myofibrils*.

• **Myofibril**: Each single Myofibril sSrand of the Muscle Fiber is made up of the smallest of all the Fiber bundles, called *Myofilaments*. Muscular Contraction occurs here.

• **Myosin** and **Actin**: Within each Myofilament are the Contractile Proteins, Myosin and Actin, which are the smallest moving parts of the Muscle.

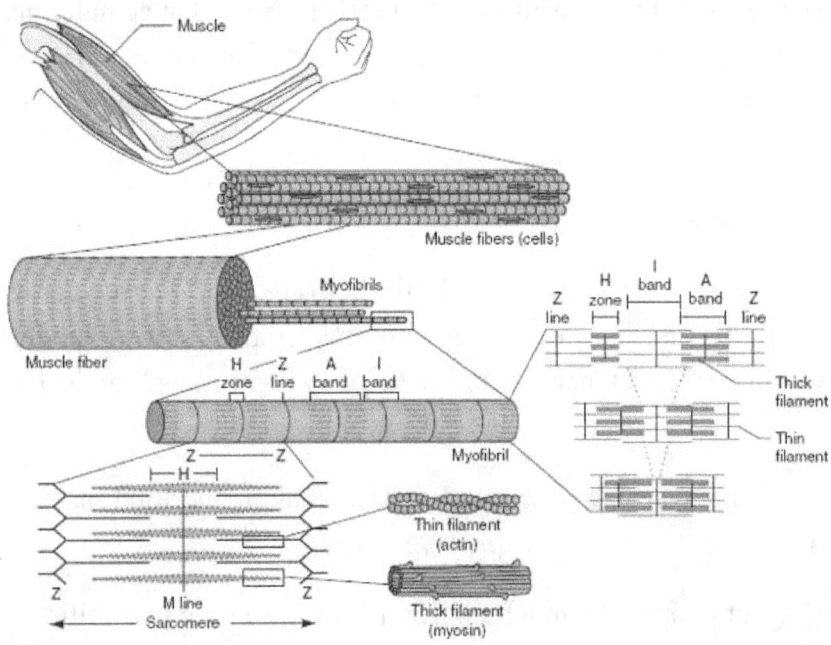

Muscle Action

Inside the Muscle Fiber, structures run the length of the Cell that are called *Myofibrils*. Myofibrils contain the Contractile Proteins, Myosin and Actin, which interact in the presence of Calcium to **shorten** the Cell (and the Muscle). The Muscle shortens to **cause Movement** in different directions at the Joint. When the Calcium is **pumped-out** of the surrounding fluid, the Cell then **relaxes** to return the Muscle elastically to its Resting Length.

This alternating process of Muscle Contraction and Relaxation can continue until Muscle Glycogen is **depleted** and Muscle Fatigue occurs.

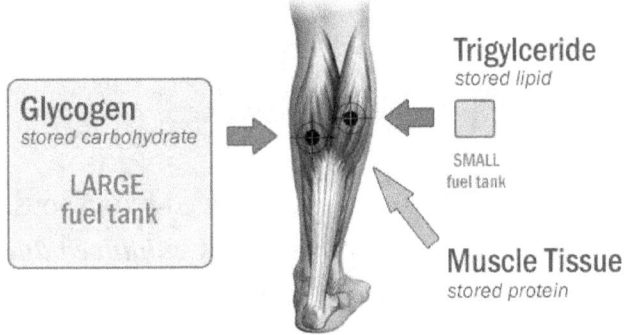

Fuel Sources

Fuel sources at rest are a mix of Carbohydrate and Fat. During exercise, the Carbohydrate is the **primary fuel**, and with **longer** Aerobic bouts, some Fat is used, which equates to Fat 'burning' or loss.

A fuel of last resort is protein, which is only used when the other fuels are exhausted.

The High-Energy compound that manifest Life Energy to our Body Cells is Adenosine Tri-Phosphate (ATP), the Energy currency of the Cell.

Various forms of Energy are called on for successive energy needs:

• **Immediate Energy**: High-power or immediate Energy demands over a short time depend on ATP being readily available within the Muscle Tissue. This amount is used rapidly, and a backup compound, Creatine Phosphate (CP), is made available. These High-Energy compounds, however, will sustain exercise for only **5 to 8 seconds**.

• **Short-term Energy**: For Anaerobic bursts like sprints and weight lifting (between 30 seconds and 2 minutes), Muscle Glycogen provides the **only** available Fuel source through the Lactate Pathway. Although the amount of available Glycogen is small, it is an **important rapid** source of Energy for **brief** Muscular effort.

• **Long-term Energy**: Exercise continuing more than 2 minutes requires an significant Oxygen-dependent, or Aerobic, Energy system. A **constant** supply of Oxygen in the Blood is necessary for continued exercise. The Mitochondria, which are Organelles within the Cell, produce large amounts of ATP. The ATP is produced mainly from Glucose and Fatty Acids and supplies the continued Energy needs of the body.

Energy During Exercise

For activities lasting **less** than 1 hour, most athletes do not need Exogenous sources of Energy during the exercise period. **However, performance is enhanced during longer endurance events with the interval consumption of Carbohydrates**. The American College of Sports Medicine, the Academy of Nutrition and Dietetics (formerly American Dietetic Association), and the Dietitians of Canada **recommend** eating or drinking 0.7 g of Carbs **per** kilogram of body weight **per** hour (approximately 30 to 60 g/hour) during long events. **The food of choice should provide Carbohydrates primarily from Glucose, with little or no Fat, Protein, or Fiber**.

Energy After Exercise: Recovery

Proper Nutrition is not only important to the athlete before and during exercise, but it also plays a major role in **recovery** after the event. It is well accepted that Fluid and Carbohydrates consumed **within 30 minutes** after a Glycogen-depleting endurance event will result in better Glycogen **synthesis** and Muscle **recovery** than if those same replacement nutrients were consumed 2 hours or more after the event.

Beverages of 6% Glucose concentration are adequate during this period, but higher concentrations may be consumed, depending on the tolerance of the athlete.

For athletes recovering for longer periods of time, a replacement meal or beverage containing 1.2 g of carbohydrate per kilogram of body weight (over several hours) results in an increased rate of Muscle Glycogen recovery.

Classification of Exercise Intensity

Intensity	% Max Heart Rate	%VO₂ Max	Perceived Exertion
Light	57-63	37-45	Very light to fairly light
Moderate	64-76	46-63	Fairly light to somewhat hard
Vigorous	77-95	64-90	Somewhat hard to very hard

• As part of their *60 or more minutes* of **daily** physical activity, children and adolescents should include muscle-strengthening physical activity on at **least 3 days** of the week.

• As part of their **60 or more minutes** of **daily** physical activity, children and adolescents should include Bone-strengthening physical activity on at least **3 days of the week**.

*Adults: **Avoid inactivity***. Some physical activity is better than none, and adults who participate in any amount of physical activity gain some health benefits.

• For substantial health benefits, adults should do at **least 150 minutes** (2 hours and 30 minutes) a week of **moderate-intensity**, or **75 minutes** (1 hour and 15 minutes) a week of **vigorous-intensity** Aerobic physical activity, or an equivalent combination of moderate- and vigorous-intensity Aerobic activity.

Aerobic activity should be performed in episodes of *at least 10 minutes*, and preferably, it should be spread throughout the week.

• For additional and more extensive Health benefits, adults should *increase* their Aerobic physical activity to *300 minutes* (5 hours) a week of *moderate-intensity*, or *150 minutes a week* of *vigorous-intensity* Aerobic physical activity, or an *equivalent combination* of moderate- and vigorous-intensity activity.

Additional health benefits are gained by engaging in physical activity beyond this amount.

• Adults should also do Muscle-Strengthening activities that are *moderate or high-intensity* and involve ALL major Muscle groups on at least *2 or more days a week*, as these activities provide *additional* Health benefits.

Older Adults: The guidelines for adults also apply to older adults. In addition, the following guidelines are just for older adults:

• When older adults *cannot* do at least *150 minutes* of *moderate-intensity* Aerobic activity a week because of chronic conditions, they should be as physically active as their abilities and conditions allow.

• Older adults should do exercises that *maintain* or *improve* Balance if they are at risk of falling.

• Older adults should determine their level of effort for physical activity relative to their level of fitness.

• Older adults with chronic conditions should understand *whether* and *how* their conditions affect their ability to do regular physical activity safely.

Myths and Misinformation

Athletes and their coaches are particularly susceptible to myths and claims about foods and dietary supplements, relentlessly searching for the competitive edge.

Knowing this, marketers unremittingly exploit this hunt.

Manufacturers sometimes make ***distorted*** and ***false*** claims about products. For an example, Pangamic Acid was ***marketed*** as "vitamin B_{15}," although it is ***not*** a vitamin at all and carried claims about its ability to enhance oxygen transport during exercise, to lessen muscle fatigue, and to increase endurance.

Naturally, if such a compound existed, then it would be of interest to athletes and their trainers.

However, scientific research has exposed these claims as unfounded.

Nevertheless, products and advertisements still appear for "vitamin B_{15}," although it is currently illegal to distribute pangamic acid in the United States.

EFT Heart & Soul
The AMT 2012
www.TheAMT.com

EFT

Emotional
Freedom
Techniques

Top of the head

Third Eye point
Eyebrow point
Corner of the eye
Under eye

Under nose

Under mouth

Under Collarbone

Thumb
Index Finger
Middle Finger
Ring Finger
Little Finger

*Start and finish
by placing both
hands flat on the
centre of the chest,
and take 3 deep
breaths in and out.*

Karate Chop Point

"What is causing you stress today?"

Critical Thinking

1.   If I help YOU to Eliminate YOUR Causes of Death ... What are YOU left with??

2.   How Long Do You Want To Live??

Chapter 10 ...

Science of Self-Healing!

*****

The Human Body is Created to literally Heal itself. This might seem to be an obvious statement, because we are well aware that wounds *heal* and Cells routinely *replace* themselves. Nonetheless, this is a profound concept because Self-Healing is the basis of *ALL* Healing.

External manipulations simply mobilize the body's *Inner* Healing Resources.

Instead of focusing on why the Body's Cells are sick, I ask WHY the body is not *replacing its* sick *Cells with* healthy *Cells.*

The body's ability to be well or ill is largely tied to inner resources, and the external environment—social and physical—has an impact on this ability.

What is the evidence for self-healing? The long and common history of clinical observations of the "placebo effect," the "laying on of hands," or "spontaneous remissions" may be included in this category.

In paraphrasing Carl Jung: Summoned or unsummoned, self-healing will be there. Self-healing is so powerful that biomedical methodology mainly designs double-blind, controlled clinical trials to see what percentage of benefit powerful drugs can add to the healing encounter.

Another related concept is that the body has Energy which I cover in another work entitled – 'Understanding Our Human Energy Systems: Energy Cycles & Transformations to Achieve Abundant Life!'.

Accordingly, as a living entity, the Body is an Energetic system. Disruptions in the *Balance* and *Flow* of this Energy is the root cause illness, and the body's *response* to Energetic imbalance leads to perceptible dis-ease.

Everything is ATOMS – including Us. Atoms are Energy based elements, so focusing on and finding Energy-based Solutions are the most effective and Successful endeavors.

Because the Body heals itself, the Body can also make itself sick. Restoring or facilitating the Body to restore its own Balance is the catalyst for restoring Health.

The symptoms of a cold, flu, or allergy are caused by the Body's efforts to *rid* itself of the offending agent. For an example, by raising the body's temperature, a fever reduces bacterial reproduction (like an antibiotic, fever is literally bacteriostatic), and sneezing physically expels offending agents.

Our Bodies are designed to keep us here for a very long time. Our Breathing, Hydration and Energy/food intake are the formula for dis-ease and pre-mature death or the Successful Enjoyment of Abundant Life!

Relaxation Exercises

An effective relaxation technique is anything that helps reduce sensory overload by redirecting positive sensations through the five senses. However, just like throwing a football, building with wood, or sewing, it is a skill and must be practiced for an individual to be good at it

Meditation

Herbert Benson in his book *The Relaxation Response* describes a useful form of meditation. The components include the following:

Relaxation Response - Reversal of Stress symptoms.

■   *Quiet* room with *minimal* distractions.

■   A *comfortable* sitting position with most of the body weight supported to *avoid* muscular tension or falling asleep.

■ A **Focus** word or phrase used to **replace** all other thoughts. It can be a repetition of a mantra that should invoke Peace and Tranquility in Self. This exercise can seem monotonous, but it will **clear** your Mind of unnecessary mental clutter and chatter.

■ **Passive attitude**. Disregard distracting thoughts or concerns. Any time your attention drifts, simply say, **"no" or "Oh, well"** to yourself and **return** to silently repeating your Focus word or phrase.

■ **Proper breathing**. Oxygen is the Breath Of Life in Atomic form. It is the ONE Life function that we MUST perform properly. As you Inhale through your Nose, you should feel your Lungs **fill** completely and your belly **expand** fully. As you Exhale through your Nose, your belly will fall.

A Session involves keeping your eyes **closed** and **slowly** Inhaling and Exhaling. At the end of each exhalation, mentally say the mantra (e.g., the word *one* or *peace*).

When you first Start, go for 10 minutes. Gradually **add** time until a session is approximately 20 minutes daily, preferably at a specific time each day.

Progressive Muscle Relaxation

Muscle Tension is the most common symptom of Stress, but where each of us feels it varies. One woman might have a tight neck and shoulders, while another feels an iron band digging into her forehead. It is not always easy to locate and relax the muscles responsible.

Progressive Muscle Relaxation (PMR) teaches you to **isolate** specific sets of Muscles, **tense** them briefly, and then **relax** them.

This exercise is especially helpful if your Mind is racing, making it hard to settle down to other techniques.

What's the Science...

Progressive Muscular Relaxation

Systematically Tensing and Relaxing the body's Muscles from the Feet to the Head.

It takes only about 10 minutes to exercise all the major body areas. There are several sequences.

You can start with the hand muscles, progressing to others; begin at the top, moving from head to toe; or reverse the direction, going from bottom to top as explained here:

PMR Procedure

Find a comfortable position. Perform the steps while either sitting or lying down, preferably in a quiet, soothing environment.

Breathe deeply, allowing your Stomach to *rise* as you Inhale and *fall* as you Exhale. Breathe this way for a few minutes before starting.

For *each* of the Body areas, perform *three* contractions:

■   First contraction: 100% intensity for 5 to 10 seconds

■   Release and relax (exhale)

■   Compare relaxation to contraction

■   Second contraction: 50% intensity for 5 to 10 seconds

■   Release and relax (exhale)

■   Compare relaxation to contraction

■   Third contraction: 5% to 10% intensity for 5 to 10 seconds

■   Release and relax (exhale)

■   Compare relaxation to contraction

Take your time, *slowly* working through *each* of these Body areas:

1. *Curl* Toes tightly.

2. *Flex* the Feet.

3. *Tighten* the Calves.

4. *Tense* the Thighs.

5. *Tighten* the Buttocks.

6. *Tighten* the Lower Back.

7. *Tighten* the Abdomen.

8. *Tense* the Upper Chest.

9. *Tense* the Upper Back Muscles.

10. *Clench* the Fists.

11. *Extend* the Fingers and flex the Wrists.

12. *Tighten* the Forearms.

13. *Tighten* the Upper Arms.

14. *Lift* the Shoulders gently toward the ears.

15. *Wrinkle* the Forehead.

16. *Squeeze* your Eyes shut.

17. *Drop* your Chin, letting your Mouth open wide.

Prayer

Prayer is one of the oldest and most commonly used methods of *coping* with Life problems.

 If you are Spiritual or Religious, Prayer WILL *promote* Mental and Physical health.

A Prayer commonly associated with stress seeks Divine *guidance* or Divine *intervention*.

Such Prayers are used when you need help yourself or when you Pray for help to be given to others.

Mental Imagery

Imagination will produce Feelings of Relaxation. For example, Visualize yourself feeling Warm, Calm, and Relaxed.

IT'S JUST THAT EASY TO CONTROL YOUR OWN EMOTIONAL WELL-BEING!

Now Picture a Tranquil setting that appeals to you and *create* a Mental *picture* of the details.

Visualize *tranquil* Mental images to *relax* you when you are Stressed.

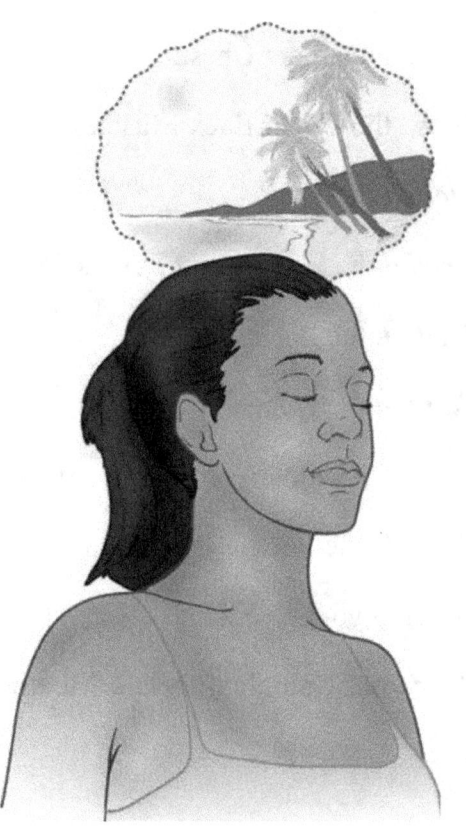

■   *Mental imagery* is generating images that have a Calming, Healing effect.

■   *Visualization* is Mental Imagery consciously directed by yourself.

■   In *Guided Mental Imagery*, *images* are suggested by another person, either live or on tape.

Mental imagery can be used in a stressful situation (e.g., before making a public speech, at the start of an exam, while waiting in line, while sitting in a dentist's chair, during a meeting).

The technique can also be used to change your habits or improve your performance in various activities. Visualize, or imagine, yourself doing something differently or performing successfully.

Visualize YourSelf Enjoying Abundant Life ……. OPEN YOUR EYES AND MAKE IT REALITY!!!!!

Life Energy Exercise

Yoga

Based on traditional Indian philosophy, Yoga is an excellent way to *invigorate* the Body and simultaneously *calm* the Mind. There are many different types of Yoga, with each sharing certain basic or core elements: Pranayamas (rhythmic breathing), Meditation, and Asanas (stretching postures).

One of the most commonly practiced forms is Hatha Yoga, which has relatively gentle movements that can be tailored to your ability. Like Tai Chi and Qi Gong, yoga *increases* Flexibility and Coordination while *releasing* Muscle Tension, and *enhancing* Tranquility.

Asanas - Various postures used in doing yoga exercises.

Tai Chi

Tai chi, a series of slow, fluid, circular motions, originated as a martial art. Its low-intensity movements produce declines in blood pressure similar to those achieved with *moderate-intensity* Aerobics.

Qi Gong

Qi Gong is a blend of **breathing**, **meditation**, **gentle exercise**, and **flowing movements**. When practiced regularly, it can **lower** Blood Pressure, Pulse, and demand for Oxygen.

Rhythmic, Repetitive Activities

Rhythmic exercises, such as **walking**, **jogging**, **swimming**, or **bicycling**, can be **calming** and **relaxing**. *Use a passive attitude and when disruptive thoughts intrude, gently turn your mind away from them and focus on moving and breathing rhythmically.*

Massage

Research indicates that Human touch is **vital** for Well-being. For an example, infants **require** Human touch to **thrive**. People of all ages need it as well.

All forms of massage tend to be both **relaxing** and **invigorating**. Massage requires the assistance of someone else to achieve full benefit.

Hydrotherapy (e.g., baths, hot tubs, jacuzzis, saunas) is another form of muscle massage.

Going Above and Beyond

Websites

American Institute of Stress

http://www.stress.org

American Psychological Association

http://www.apa.org http://www.apa.org/helpcenter/index.aspx

The Humor Project

http://www.humorproject.com

National Institute for Occupational Safety and Health (NIOSH)

http://www.cdc.gov/niosh/stresshp.html

National Institute of Mental Health

http://www.nimh.nih.gov

National Sleep Foundation

http://www.sleepfoundation.org

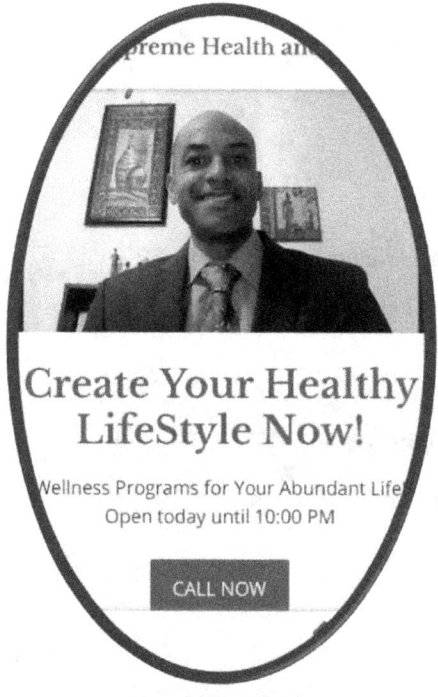

Chapter 11 ...

The Sum Up!

*****

The Energy Molecule of the Body is ATP, and the Powerhouse of the Cell is the Mitochondrion. We are comprised of TRILLIONS of these Cells. The Cell's **depot** of Energy is Creatine Phosphate. These two High-Energy Phosphate compounds are in significantly **limited** supply. They can produce or make manifest Energy for a **brief initial period only** and **need to be replenished** for exercise to continue.

This added supply is produced or manifested by Anaerobic Glycolysis, with Energy made available for **continued** exercise by the body's Aerobic system. The process of Glycolysis metabolizes only the Carbohydrate Substrate, which is furnished by either Blood Glucose or stored Glycogen.

Dietary Carbs is necessary to **replenish** these necessary Fuel sources.

Protein contributes little to Energy for exercise, whereas the body's ability to 'burn' Fat as fuel depends on the **level** *of fitness and* **intensity** *of exercise.*

The higher the Body's efficiency in using Oxygen, the more fatty acids will contribute to the energy supply = MORE ADIPOSE FAT TISSUE LOSS!

We are Oxygen dependent and the 1ˢᵗ or Major benefit for exercising is Increase in Oxygen in-take = Maximum Oxygenation. This is the foundation to Successfully Build YOUR Own Supreme Health and Fitness and the catalyst to Enjoying Abundant Life!

Even in the best-trained athletes, Fatty Acid Oxidation (Fat/Weight loss) must be accompanied by Glucose Metabolism.

Contrary to popular belief (which is an advertising invention), exercise does not require an increased in-take of Vitamins or Minerals.

The body's increased needs are well supplied by a *normal healthy diet*. Exercise *increases* the body's *need* for KCalories and Water.

Drink Luke-warm, room-temperature water in small, frequent amounts is the best way to *prevent* dehydration in *most athletic events and exercise*.

In most cases, Electrolytes lost in sweat are replaced by a diet of adequate quality and quantity.

A mild Saline and Glucose solution (4% to 8%) may supply *fluid* and *fuel* to sustain Energy during *longer endurance events*.

Some athletes use *harmful* practices such as food and fluid deprivation for controlling weight, as well as such Ergogenic aids as illegal steroid drugs for bulking muscles.

The health benefits of general and aerobic exercise are numerous. Excellent aerobic exercises include *sustained fast walking*, *swimming*, *jogging*, *running*, and *aerobic dancing or workouts*.

<u>*Approach any exercise sensibly, and choose those activities that are enjoyable.*</u>

Childhood to Abundant Life!

If you expect to become a parent, bear this in mind: The *Ability of becoming able to Successfully Enjoy Abundant Life starts with a physically active life that begins in childhood.*

You will do your children no favors if you allow them to watch television or play computer games most of the time. Encourage children to Balance those activities with sports, games, or other physical activity that they enjoy.

As children become LESS physically active, the Natural Life Energy is diminishing, and dis-eases that normally affect adults is INCREASING in children.

OBESITY AND DIABETES (and the detrimental Health issues) are manifesting in adolescents and pre-teens !

Also, remember that as a parent you are a model for your child. Take time to do activities with your children to encourage them to spend time exercising.

Continue to exercise as you age. You'll have a *healthier* Heart and Fitter Body.

Constant and Consistent Exercise will significantly *reduce* Blood Pressure, make your Joints more *flexible*, and *increase* Muscular *strength* and *endurance*.

Not only your body benefits: You will improve your mood and your cognitive functions as well.

Keeping your balance as you age is a major issue. Falls that a young person bounces back from can incapacitate or be fatal for older people. Falls in old age are usually the result of poor balance, and keeping fit improves balance.

Even if you did not start early – Yesterday …… You can start late- Today….. RIGHT NOW!!!!!!!!!!

IT'S NEVER TOO LATE!!!!!!

All it akes is for YOU to make the Decision…..Decide on Life……Decide HOW Long YOU Want to Live …… Put this Book DOWN, GET UP AND GO DO IT!!!

YES, IT IS THIS EASY!

Enjoying Abundant Life!

PEACE

Sean Ali,

Facts & Figures

*****

Steps in Decision Making

After reading this book, I pray that you are able to realize how important it is to make the necessary decision for Beginning and Maintaining a healthy lifestyle.

To make good decisions, you can use the following procedures.

1.   **Identify and clarify the problem.** You must recognize that a problem exists. Some may simply be annoyances, while others are big issues.

2.   **Gather information.** Learn more about the problem situation. Look for possible causes and solutions.

3.   **Evaluate the evidence.** How accurate is the information? Is it fact or opinion?

4.   **Consider alternatives and implications.** Draw conclusions, then weigh the advantages and disadvantages of each alternative.

5.   **Choose and implement the best alternative.**

These procedures apply to any of life's decisions, not merely those dealing with a healthy lifestyle.

Exercise Myths or Misconceptions

Misconceptions exist about what is exercise fact and what is exercise fiction. Here are some common exercise-related fallacies:

■   Passive muscle stimulators expend Energy from the electrical outlet in the wall, *not* from your Cells. ***The Energy expended to bring about Fat loss must be from* within *your Body.***

■   Taking a pill to bring about instant changes in fitness is an ***illusion***. ***Fitness takes time and effort***. The body systems (muscular, cardiovascular, and skeletal) become ***stronger*** in response to ***regular physical activity.***

■   ***<u>Cellulite</u> is not something a health gadget or cream can eliminate. Rapid*** gain or loss of body Fat causes the dimpled look associated with the term *Cellulite*.

■   Shake, rattle, or roll your Fat—*it won't disappear*. The ***only*** way to ***reduce*** body fat is to ***use more*** Energy than you ***consume*** in Calories.

■   Wearing rubberized suits, extra layers of clothing, or working out in a hot environment ***loses Body Water, not Body Fat***. It takes a ***great deal*** of Heat to melt Fat. ***Such Heat would melt the rest of you as well***.

■   If spot reduction worked, everyone who chewed gum or talked a lot would have a narrow face.

■   Exercise ***does not*** turn Body Fat Cells into Muscle Cells, ***nor does*** inactivity turn Muscle Cells into Fat. They are ***different*** types of Cells. ***Eat too much and be inactive, and you will* enlarge (<u>Hypertrophy</u>) *the Fat cClls in your body and* shrink (<u>Atrophy</u>) *the Muscle Cells***. Eat right and exercise to do the reverse.

■   Rubbing lotions on the skin to lose fat, firm up muscles, or remove Lactic Acid ***does not work***. Resistance training firms up muscles.

■   Eating ***extra*** Protein to ***build*** stronger muscles ***doesn't work***. ***When someone eats more Protein than your body uses, the extra will be stored by your body as fat***. ***Increased muscle size comes through resistance training.***

■ Losing inches is not necessarily loss of Fat. It can also be loss of Water or Lean Muscle Tissue.

■ Exercise is only tiring momentarily. It then makes you feel more energetic as you become more fit.

■ In women, Resistance Training mainly increases Muscle Strength, NOT Size.

■ Drinking liquids during exercise ***does not*** cause **cramping**. Cool water or other appropriate drinks (not soda) should be consumed before, during, and after exercising to replace lost fluids.

Evaluating the Quality of Internet Information Sources

You can find information on just about everything on the Internet. Of course, not all Internet sites are created equal. Some present research and information, some are trying to sell a product, and some are flat-out misinformation. Here are some suggestions on how to decide whether the information you find is quality and reputable:

1. **Check for the creator of the site.** It is important to be able to identify whom the authors or creators of the site are. The author should include his or her credentials to demonstrate his or her training and expertise in the subject matter. If this information is missing, be cautious.

2. **Check the URL.** Website addresses that end with .edu are material from an educational or research institution. Those ending in .gov are government sources. Those ending with .com or .biz are commercial sites generally intended to sell a product. Because the content of websites is not monitored for accuracy, you may be reading inaccurate, biased, misleading, partial, or false information. This is much more likely to occur on commercial sites than on any other type of website. In addition, if the URL includes a personal name, the site may simply be an individual creating a forum for his or her personal opinion.

3. **Check for advertising.** Websites often accept advertising to help pay the cost of maintaining the site. If the products being advertised are the same as or related to the nature of the information you seek, be cautious.

You'd hate to rely on information that has been biased so as not to offend or upset an advertiser. When that happens, you can be certain the information you are viewing is misleading.

4. **Look for accuracy.** Be on the lookout for sites that integrate personal opinions, testimonials, or leading statements about the material you are searching for. Do not assume the first site you visit has accurate information. Gather information from several sites on the same topic and look for common themes. Sites that go into greater depth with their information (as opposed to stating one "fact" and then presenting opinion afterward) are more likely to be accurate. Always back up data from Internet sources with other forms of information to make your data gathering more comprehensive and, in turn, more accurate.

5. **Look for timeliness.** Websites should always contain "updated on" dates to indicate when the information was created. If these dates are missing, you should find additional sources to support the materials' timeliness. Some websites are created but then never updated, and there is no systematic removal of old sites from the Internet. In addition, many sites contain links to other websites or other information. If many of the links are no longer available or contain outdated material, exercise caution regarding what you find. Make certain you find supporting materials from other sources.

Identifying Fitness Misinformation and Quackery

Some advertisers claim—*mostly without evidence*—that their fitness products offer a quick, easy way to shape up, keep fit, and lose weight. *There is no such thing as a no-work, no-sweat way to a healthy, fit body. To get the benefit, you have to do the work.*

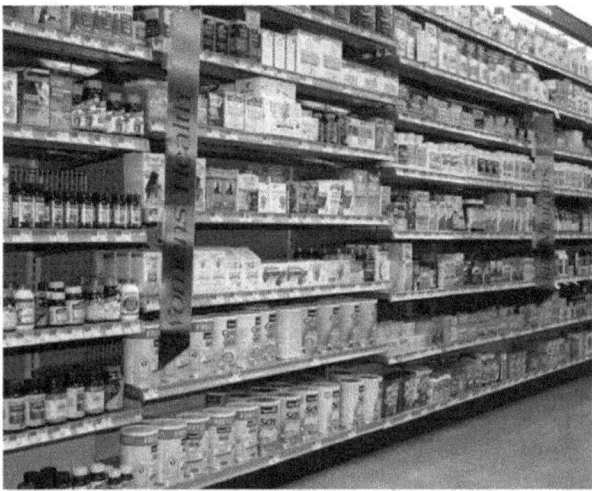

Watch for these and other warning signs:

■   If the claim sounds too good to be true, it probably is.

■   If a product really worked, you would see it in headlines, not just in ads.

■   The ads claim the product treats a wide range of ailments.

■   The information given is unclear, vague, and highly emotional.

■   Changes are promised to be quick, dramatic, or miraculous.

■   Results are promised to be easy, effortless, guaranteed, or permanent.

■   The ads claim relief from conditions for which there are few treatments and no cures.

■   The promoter blames problems on a build-up of toxins in the body.

■   Ads declare the medical community to be against the discovery.

■   The ads rely on a guru, testimonials, case histories, and before-and-after photos.

■   Products are sold door-to-door, in fliers, through pop-up ads, or by mail order and television advertisements.

■   The promoter uses high-pressure sales tactics, one-time-only deals, recruitment for a pyramid sales organization, or demands for large advance payments or long-term contracts.

Choosing Supplements

The next time you watch a TV commercial or see a flyer for a quick weight-loss program, take a moment to consider it. What is being said to you? Who is saying it? In today's day and age we find that to be healthy consumers we need to be educated consumers. The next time you see one of these ads, take a minute to answer the following questions:

■   What claim is being made on behalf of this product?

■   Who is making this claim? Is it an outside source or the company that makes the product?

■   Is everything a testimony about how miraculous the product is?

■   Does the ad list any studies that have been done to demonstrate the product's effectiveness?

■   If yes, is this a credible source?

■   Does it seem like a miracle cure or solution?

■   How does it make you feel that ineffective or dangerous products may be marketed without any sound research?

Reflect * Reinforce * Reinvigorate

Dietary Reference Intakes (DRIs)

Dietary Reference Intakes (DRIs): Recommended Dietary Allowances and Adequate Intakes, Vitamins

Life Stage Group	Vitamin A (µg/d)[a]	Vitamin C (mg/d)	Vitamin D (µg/d)[b,c]	Vitamin E (mg/d)[d]	Vitamin E (mg/d)[d]	Thiamin (mg/d)	Riboflavin (mg/d)	Niacin (mg/d)[e]	Vitamin B$_6$ (mg/d)	Folate (µg/d)[f]	Vitamin B$_{12}$ (µg/d)	Pantothenic Acid (m	Biotin (µg/d)	Choline (mg/d)[g]
Infants														
0–6 mo	400*	40*	10	4*	2.0*	0.2*	0.3*	2*	0.1*	65*	0.4*	1.7*	5*	125*
6–12 mo	500*	50*	10	5*	2.5*	0.3*	0.4*	4*	0.3*	80*	0.5*	1.8*	6*	150*
Children														
1–3 y	300	15	15	6	30*	0.5	0.5	6	0.5	150	0.9	2*	8*	200*
4–8 y	400	25	15	7	55*	0.6	0.6	8	0.6	200	1.2	3*	12*	250*
Males														
9–13 y	600	45	15	11	60*	0.9	0.9	12	1.0	300	1.8	4*	20*	375*
14–18 y	900	75	15	15	75*	1.2	1.3	16	1.3	400	2.4	5*	25*	550*
19–30 y	900	90	15	15	120*	1.2	1.3	16	1.3	400	2.4	5*	30*	550*
31–50 y	900	90	15	15	120*	1.2	1.3	16	1.3	400	2.4	5*	30*	550*
51–70 y	900	90	15	15	120*	1.2	1.3	16	1.7	400	2.4[h]	5*	30*	550*
>70 y	900	90	20	15	120*	1.2	1.3	16	1.7	400	2.4[h]	5*	30*	550*
Females														
9–13 y	600	45	15	11	60*	0.9	0.9	12	1.0	300	1.8	4*	20*	375*
14–18 y	700	65	15	15	75*	1.0	1.0	14	1.2	400[i]	2.4	5*	25*	400*
19–30 y	700	75	15	15	90*	1.1	1.1	14	1.3	400[i]	2.4	5*	30*	425*
31–50 y	700	75	15	15	90*	1.1	1.1	14	1.3	400[i]	2.4	5*	30*	425*
51–70 y	700	75	15	15	90*	1.1	1.1	14	1.5	400	2.4[h]	5*	30*	425*
>70 y	700	75	20	15	90*	1.1	1.1	14	1.5	400	2.4[h]	5*	30*	425*
Pregnancy														
14–18 y	750	80	15	15	75*	1.4	1.4	18	1.9	600[j]	2.6	6*	30*	450*
19–30 y	770	85	15	15	90*	1.4	1.4	18	1.9	600[j]	2.6	6*	30*	450*
31–50 y	770	85	15	15	90*	1.4	1.4	18	1.9	600[j]	2.6	6*	30*	450*
Lactation														
14–18 y	1,200	115	15	19	75*	1.4	1.6	17	2.0	500	2.8	7*	35*	550*
19–30 y	1,300	120	15	19	90*	1.4	1.6	17	2.0	500	2.8	7*	35*	550*
31–50 y	1,300	120	15	19	90*	1.4	1.6	17	2.0	500	2.8	7*	35*	550*

Dietary Reference Intakes (DRIs): Tolerable Upper Intake Levels, Vitamins

Life Stage Group	Vitamin A (µg/d)[a]	Vitamin C (mg/d)	Vitamin D (µg/d)	Vitamin E (mg/d)[b,c]	Vitamin K	Thiamin	Riboflavin	Niacin (mg/d)[c]	Vitamin B6 (mg/d)	Folate (µg/d)[c]	Vitamin B12	Pantothenic Acid	Biotin	Choline (g/d)	Carotenoids[d]
Infants															
0–6 mo	600	ND[e]	25	ND	ND	ND	ND	ND	ND	ND	ND	ND	ND	ND	ND
6–12 mo	600	ND	38	ND	ND	ND	ND	ND	ND	ND	ND	ND	ND	ND	ND
Children															
1–3 y	600	400	63	200	ND	ND	ND	10	30	300	ND	ND	ND	1.0	ND
4–8 y	900	650	75	300	ND	ND	ND	15	40	400	ND	ND	ND	1.0	ND
Males															
9–13 y	1,700	1,200	100	600	ND	ND	ND	20	60	600	ND	ND	ND	2.0	ND
14–18 y	2,800	1,800	100	800	ND	ND	ND	30	80	800	ND	ND	ND	3.0	ND
19–30 y	3,000	2,000	100	1,000	ND	ND	ND	35	100	1,000	ND	ND	ND	3.5	ND
31–50 y	3,000	2,000	100	1,000	ND	ND	ND	35	100	1,000	ND	ND	ND	3.5	ND
51–70 y	3,000	2,000	100	1,000	ND	ND	ND	35	100	1,000	ND	ND	ND	3.5	ND
>70 y	3,000	2,000	100	1,000	ND	ND	ND	35	100	1,000	ND	ND	ND	3.5	ND
Females															
9–13 y	1,700	1,200	100	600	ND	ND	ND	20	60	600	ND	ND	ND	2.0	ND
14–18 y	2,800	1,800	100	800	ND	ND	ND	30	80	800	ND	ND	ND	3.0	ND
19–30 y	3,000	2,000	100	1,000	ND	ND	ND	35	100	1,000	ND	ND	ND	3.5	ND
31–50 y	3,000	2,000	100	1,000	ND	ND	ND	35	100	1,000	ND	ND	ND	3.5	ND
51–70 y	3,000	2,000	100	1,000	ND	ND	ND	35	100	1,000	ND	ND	ND	3.5	ND
>70 y	3,000	2,000	100	1,000	ND	ND	ND	35	100	1,000	ND	ND	ND	3.5	ND
Pregnancy															
14–18 y	2,800	1,800	100	800	ND	ND	ND	30	80	800	ND	ND	ND	3.0	ND
19–30 y	3,000	2,000	100	1,000	ND	ND	ND	35	100	1,000	ND	ND	ND	3.5	ND
31–50 y	3,000	2,000	100	1,000	ND	ND	ND	35	100	1,000	ND	ND	ND	3.5	ND
Lactation															
14–18 y	2,800	1,800	100	800	ND	ND	ND	30	80	800	ND	ND	ND	3.0	ND
19–30 y	3,000	2,000	100	1,000	ND	ND	ND	35	100	1,000	ND	ND	ND	3.5	ND
31–50 y	3,000	2,000	100	1,000	ND	ND	ND	35	100	1,000	ND	ND	ND	3.5	ND

NOTE: A Tolerable Upper Intake Level (UL) is the highest level of daily nutrient intake that is likely to pose no risk of adverse health effects to almost all individuals in the general population. Unless otherwise specified, the UL represents total intake from food, water, and supplements. Due to a lack of suitable data, ULs could not be established for vitamin K, thiamin, riboflavin, vitamin B12, pantothenic acid, biotin, and carotenoids. In the absence of a UL, extra caution may be warranted in consuming levels above recommended intakes. Members of the general population should be advised not to routinely exceed the UL. The UL is not meant to apply to individuals who are treated with the nutrient under medical supervision or to individuals with predisposing conditions that modify their sensitivity to the nutrient.

[a] As preformed vitamin A only.
[b] As α-tocopherol; applies to any form of supplemental α-tocopherol.
[c] The ULs for vitamin E, niacin, and folate apply to synthetic forms obtained from supplements, fortified foods, or a combination of the two.
[d] β-carotene supplements are advised only to serve as a provitamin A source for individuals at risk of vitamin A deficiency.
[e] ND = Not determinable due to lack of data of adverse effects in this age group and concern with regard to lack of ability to handle excess amounts. Source of intake should be from food only to prevent high levels of intake.

SOURCE: Reprinted with permission from Dietary Reference Intakes, 2011 by the National Academy of Sciences. Courtesy of the National Academies Press.

Dietary Reference Intakes (DRIs): Tolerable Upper Intake Levels, Elements

Life Stage Group	Arsenic[a]	Boron (mg/d)	Calcium (mg/d)	Chromium	Copper (µg/d)	Fluoride (mg/d)	Iodine (µg/d)	Iron (mg/d)	Magnesium (mg/d)[b]	Manganese (mg/d)	Molybdenum (µg/d)	Nickel (mg/d)	Phosphorus (g/d)	Selenium (µg/d)	Silicon[c]	Vanadium (mg/d)[d]	Zinc (mg/d)	Sodium (g/d)	Chloride (g/d)
Infants																			
0-6 mo	ND[e]	ND	1,000	ND	ND	0.7	ND	40	ND	ND	ND	ND	ND	45	ND	ND	4	ND	ND
6-12 mo	ND	ND	1,500	ND	ND	0.9	ND	40	ND	ND	ND	ND	ND	60	ND	ND	5	ND	ND
Children																			
1-3 y	ND	3	2,500	ND	1,000	1.3	200	40	65	2	300	0.2	3	90	ND	ND	7	1.5	2.3
4-8 y	ND	6	2,500	ND	3,000	2.2	300	40	110	3	600	0.3	3	150	ND	ND	12	1.9	2.9
Males																			
9-13 y	ND	11	3,000	ND	5,000	10	600	40	350	6	1,100	0.6	4	280	ND	ND	23	2.2	3.4
14-18 y	ND	17	3,000	ND	8,000	10	900	45	350	9	1,700	1.0	4	400	ND	ND	34	2.3	3.6
19-30 y	ND	20	2,500	ND	10,000	10	1,100	45	350	11	2,000	1.0	4	400	ND	1.8	40	2.3	3.6
31-50 y	ND	20	2,500	ND	10,000	10	1,100	45	350	11	2,000	1.0	4	400	ND	1.8	40	2.3	3.6
51-70 y	ND	20	2,000	ND	10,000	10	1,100	45	350	11	2,000	1.0	4	400	ND	1.8	40	2.3	3.6
>70 y	ND	20	2,000	ND	10,000	10	1,100	45	350	11	2,000	1.0	3	400	ND	1.8	40	2.3	3.6
Females																			
9-13 y	ND	11	3,000	ND	5,000	10	600	40	350	6	1,100	0.6	4	280	ND	ND	23	2.2	3.4
14-18 y	ND	17	3,000	ND	8,000	10	900	45	350	9	1,700	1.0	4	400	ND	ND	34	2.3	3.6
19-30 y	ND	20	2,500	ND	10,000	10	1,100	45	350	11	2,000	1.0	4	400	ND	1.8	40	2.3	3.6
31-50 y	ND	20	2,500	ND	10,000	10	1,100	45	350	11	2,000	1.0	4	400	ND	1.8	40	2.3	3.6
51-70 y	ND	20	2,000	ND	10,000	10	1,100	45	350	11	2,000	1.0	4	400	ND	1.8	40	2.3	3.6
>70 y	ND	20	2,000	ND	10,000	10	1,100	45	350	11	2,000	1.0	3	400	ND	1.8	40	2.3	3.6
Pregnancy																			
14-18 y	ND	17	3,000	ND	8,000	10	900	45	350	9	1,700	1.0	3.5	400	ND	ND	34	2.3	3.6
19-30 y	ND	20	2,500	ND	10,000	10	1,100	45	350	11	2,000	1.0	3.5	400	ND	ND	40	2.3	3.6
61-50 y	ND	20	2,500	ND	10,000	10	1,100	45	350	11	2,000	1.0	3.5	400	ND	ND	40	2.3	3.6
Lactation																			
14-18 y	ND	17	3,000	ND	8,000	10	900	45	350	9	1,700	1.0	4	400	ND	ND	34	2.3	3.6
19-30 y	ND	20	2,500	ND	10,000	10	1,100	45	350	11	2,000	1.0	4	400	ND	ND	40	2.3	3.6
31-50 y	ND	20	2,500	ND	10,000	10	1,100	45	350	11	2,000	1.0	4	400	ND	ND	40	2.3	3.6

NOTE: A Tolerable Upper Intake Level (UL) is the highest level of daily nutrient intake that is likely to pose no risk of adverse health effects to almost all individuals in the general population. Unless otherwise specified, the UL represents total intake from food, water, and supplements. Due to a lack of suitable data, ULs could not be established for vitamin K, thiamin, riboflavin, vitamin B_{12}, pantothenic acid, biotin, and carotenoids. In the absence of a UL, extra caution may be warranted in consuming levels above recommended intakes. Members of the general population should be advised not to routinely exceed the UL. The UL is not meant to apply to individuals who are treated with the nutrient under medical supervision or to individuals with predisposing conditions that modify their sensitivity to the nutrient.

[a]Although the UL was not determined for arsenic, there is no justification for adding arsenic to food or supplements.

[b]The ULs for magnesium represent intake from a pharmacological agent only and do not include intake from food and water.

[c]Although silicon has not been shown to cause adverse effects in humans, there is no justification for adding silicon to supplements.

[d]Although vanadium in food has not been shown to cause adverse effects in humans, there is no justification for adding vanadium to food and vanadium supplements should be used with caution. The UL is based on adverse effects in laboratory animals and this data could be used to set a UL for adults but not children and adolescents.

[e]ND = Not determinable due to lack of data of adverse effects in this age group and concern with regard to lack of ability to handle excess amounts. Source of intake should be from food only to prevent high levels of intake.

Aerobic Activities

For **substantial health benefits**, adults need to do at least

•   **2 hours and 30 minutes** (150 minutes) each week of **moderate-intensity*** aerobic activity,

OR

•   **1 hour and 15 minutes** (75 minutes) each week of **vigorous-intenslty*** aerobic activity,

OR

•   An **equivalent mix of moderate- and vigorous-intensity** aerobic activity.

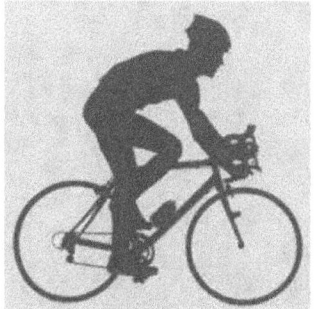

Aerobic activity should be performed for **at least 10 minutes at a time**, preferably, **spread throughout the week.**
*   **Intensity** is the level of effort required to do an activity.
     A person doing **moderate-intensity** aerobic activity can talk, but not sing, during the activity.

A person doing **vigorous-intensity** activity cannot say more than a few words without pausing for a breath.

Muscle Strengthening Activities

Muscle strengthening should be done 2 or more days a week.

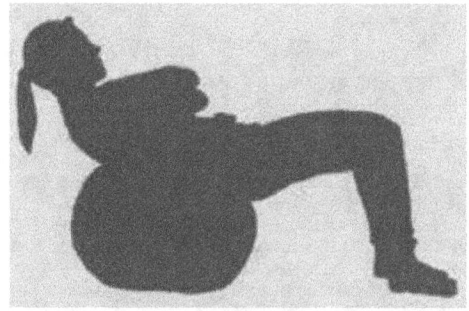

•   All major muscle groups should be worked. These are the legs, hips, back, abdomen, chest, shoulders, and arms.

•   Exercises for each muscle group should be **repeated 8 to 12** times per set. As exercises become easier, increase the weight or do another set.

How can adults get additional health benefits?

Aerobic Activities

For **greater health benefits**, adults should do

- **5 hours** (300 minutes) each week of **moderate-intensity** aerobic activity,

OR

- **2 hours and 30 minutes** (150 minutes) a week of **vigorous-intensity** aerobic activity,

OR

- An **equivalent mix of moderate- and vigorous-intensity** aerobic activity.

Health Benefits from Regular Physical Activity

Participating in regular physical activity provides many health benefits, as summarized below. Reducing risk of some of these conditions may require years of participation in regular physical activity. Other benefits, such as increased heart and lung— or cardiorespiratory—fitness, may require only a few weeks or months of participation.

Aerobic Activities by Level of Intensity

There are different ways to classify intensity of exercise. **Absolute intensity** is the amount of energy expended per minute of activity. Moderate-intensity activities expend 3.0 to 5.9 times the amount of energy expended at rest. The energy expended in vigorous-intensity activities is 6.0 or more times the energy expended at rest.

Relative intensity is the effort required for an individual to do an activity. Relative intensity of aerobic activity is related to cardiorespiratory fitness. Less fit people generally require a higher level of effort than fitter people to do the same activity. Relative intensity can be estimated using a scale of 0 to 10, where sitting is 0 and the highest level of effort possible is 10. A moderate-intensity activity is a 5 or 6. A vigorous-intensity activity is a 7 or 8.

Strong Evidence for Health Benefits

- **Lower risk of:**
  - Early death
  - Coronary heart disease
  - Stroke
  - High blood pressure
  - High cholesterol or triglycerides
  - Type 2 diabetes
  - Metabolic syndrome
  - Colon cancer
  - Breast cancer
- **Prevention of weight gain**
- **Weight loss, particularly when combined with reduced calorie intake**
- **Improved cardiorespiratory (aerobic) fitness and muscular strength**
- **Prevention of falls**
- **Reduced depression**

References and Suggested Readings

*****

Benson H. *The Relaxation Response*. New York: Avon/Wholecare, 2000.

Boscarino J. S. Diseases among men 20 years after exposure to severe stress: Implications for clinical research and medical care. *Psychosomatic Medicine* 1997; 59:605–614.

Clements K. and Turpin G. Life event exposure, physiological reactivity, and psychological strain. *Journal of Behavioral Medicine* 2000; 23:73–94.

Friedman M. and Ulmer D. *Treating Type A Behavior and Your Heart*. New York: Knopf, 1984.

Laitinen J. E., et al. Stress-related eating and drinking behavior and body-mass index and predictors of this behavior. *Preventive Medicine* 2002; 34:29–39.

McKinney C. H., et al. Effects of guided imagery and music (GIM) therapy on mood and cortisol in healthy adults. *Health Psychology* 1997; 16:390–400.

Miller M. A. and Rahe R. H. Life changes scaling for the 1990s. *Journal of Psychosomatic Research* 1997; 43:279–292.

Pashkow F. J. Is stress linked to heart disease? The evidence grows stronger. *Cleveland Clinic Journal of Medicine* 1999; 66:75–77.

Ross S., Niebling B., and Heckert T. Sources of stress among college students. *College Student Journal* 1999.

Scheufele P. M. Effects of progressive relaxation and classical music on measurements of attention, relaxation, and stress responses. *Journal of Behavioral Medicine* 2000; 23:207–228.

Seaward B. L. *Managing Stress: Principles and Strategies for Health and Wellness*, 5th ed. Sudbury, MA: Jones and Bartlett, 2006.

Selye H. *The Stress of Life*, rev. ed. New York: McGraw-Hill, 1978.

Stephens T. Physical activity and mental health in the United States and Canada: Evidence from four population surveys. *Preventive Medicine* 1988; 17:35–47.

Steptoe A. M. and Joekes K. Task demands and the pressures of everyday life: Associations between cardiovascular reactivity and work blood pressure and heart rate. *Healthy Psychology* 2000; 19:46–54.

Williams R. and Williams V. *Anger Kills*. New York: HarperCollins, 1993.

www.ingramcontent.com/pod-product-compliance
Lightning Source LLC
Chambersburg PA
CBHW081112180526
45170CB00008B/2812